The Blue Fountain

Bathing in light

Irmgard Maria Gräf

The Blue Fountain

Theory and potential of the Blu Room® technology

December 2018
Cover: Birgit Müller
Editing: Marion Collenberg

© 2018
Production and publishing: BoD - Books on Demand,
Norderstedt.
ISBN 978-3-748100140

Content

Preface

Blu Room is an extraordinary creation of light, sound, frequency and majestic architecture. Blu Room is a gift for self-healing and discovery. Here we can discover the deeper causes of our illnesses, we can perceive them attentively and lovingly and begin to heal.

The Blu Room is much more than light therapy. It affects the body, the DNA and all body fluids. It will help us to heal mind, heart and soul. Thus the Blu Room is a companion for every human being and can help them on their way to heal themselves – physically or mentally. Ultimately, we are all made of the same material and share the same essence. Until today these aspects have been neglected in medicine for healing.

 "What is the bridge?" I asked Irmgard Gräf when we first talked about Blu Room and DNA. From this first moment I recognized her genius and knew that she would get to the bottom of this question with her heart, mind and soul. In this book she introduces this invisible bridge, the medium that liberates from diseases, problems and worries.

Blu Room is where the gold meets the blue.
Blu Room is where dreams become reality.

Dr. Matthew Martinez
Co-developer of Blu Room® technology

Human life begins with fireworks

Tension! The heart races, blood vessels swell, the pulse rate rises. A male sperm meets a female ovum. The two are destined for each other. The code matches. Around 200,000 mitochondria, the small energy power plants, run at full speed in the ovum.

The tension grows. The potassium-sodium pump starts and the blood-brain barrier opens. Endorphins flow out and set the pace for a happy union. A grandiose fireworks display, triggered by 600 billion zinc atoms, announces the fusion of the male with the female egg cell. The cell lights up and proudly presents the foundation of a new life in the form of an omnipotent stem cell.

Done! Following a wonderful direction, the stem cell divides and migrates as an embryo to its new nest in the uterus. Now it's time to 'take root'. The egg membranes begin to form amniotic fluid. Soon the tiny embryo floats in a ball of protective, cuddly warm amniotic fluid, like in its own mini ocean.

Amniotic fluid is the first protected atmosphere of the young embryo. It is a field of becoming and growing in love, acceptance and timelessness. It breathes in it and performs wonderful movements - unencumbered by a world with all its possible challenges and potentials.

These pictures of the amniotic mini ocean lead me back to one of my early Blu Room experiences.

The door locks gently, music waves fill the octogonal room, my back sinks into the padded couch and the mirror surfaces absorb my restlessness. My eyelids close, my chest lifts and lowers with the breath. The ultra violet light embraces me. I am hardly aware of the music and my breathing calms down.

A deep relaxation flows through my body. Like in the amniotic fluid I feel in resonance with life, protected and carried by love and benevolence. The daily workloads, the many chores and everything on my long "to do" list suddenly lose their challenge. My outer peace is an expression of my inner balance.

Is an atom visible?

Molecules are made up of atoms.

Cells are made up of molecules.

Humans consist of cells.

Is man visible?

If you change an atom, you change the human being.

Welcome to the world of quantum physics.

This book *The Blue Fountain* takes us on a journey to discover the hidden workings of the Blu Room. We meet secrets of life and creation - and recognize ourselves as creative beings in them.

I refer to the many scientific explanations and detailed background information in the master book: *Blu Room - Experience the Future.* (1)

In this book, *The Blue Fountain*, we will encounter the invisible at every turn. This will be done in an easily recognizable and measurable fashion.

Bathing in the sun

Sunbathing Creatures

The mythical sunbird Caladrius
An early Christian theory of nature describes Caladrius as a pure white bird. It gives him the reputation of a prophetic, swan-like creature that heals all diseases and is at home both in the sun and in the ruling dynasties. The Caladrius can heal. If a person is seriously ill, the bird is called. Should the bird look away, it is a sign of inevitable death. But when he looks into the eyes of the sick person, he takes his illness and flies with it to the sun. The sun, so the myths say, burns and destroys the disease.

The sunbather, the Chinese nightingale
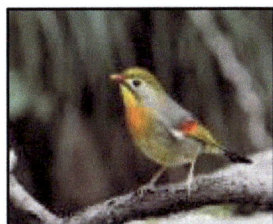
The sunbird with its bright yellow plumage owes its name to its hunger for the sun. It likes to take extensive sunbaths in large containers and widely spread his plumage. His beautiful, uniquely imaginative singing brings joy to the heart. He is also known as a Chinese nightingale.

Radiant Sun Animals
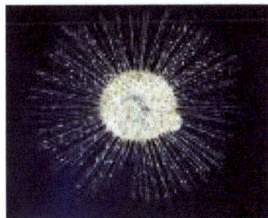
The spherical sun-animals (Heliozoa) are unicellular beings. They are beautiful, very delicate microorganisms. From a small, spherical core, thin pseudopods are stretched out in all directions, which are reinforced with so-called axopodia, which are axial threads. These can be melted down at lightning speed in case of disturbances and can then be formed again. A sun animal cannot lose its rays due to mechanical influences.

Majestic sunflowers

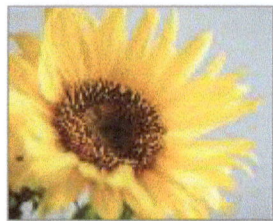 The sunflower originates from Central America, Peru and Mexico. In its homeland it is regarded as a symbol of the sun god and his male power. Majestically it wears his unfolded crown of rays on the up to 5 m high stem.

Symbolically, it strengthens the spine both physically and metaphorically and helps all those who need more assertiveness. In its clarity it stands for mature individuality, for personal strength and strong charisma. Aztec priestesses wear crowns of sunflowers as a symbol of fertility, health and wisdom.

Young sunflowers await the sunrise with their petals facing east. In this way they catch the first rays of the sun, warm up faster and attract their pollinators. The young flower follows the course of the sun to the west. At night it swings back to the east. Once the sunflower has grown up and the flower is wide open, overall growth slows down. She begins to store sun and life energy to strengthen the seed of the next season.

Sun bathing and sun healing

Since time immemorial, people have been fascinated by the radiant ball of the sun in the sky, without it no life would be possible here on our planet. In all cultures the sun is worshipped as divine, primarily as a giver of light, warmth, power, then of course also as a sign of confidence, continuity, hope, as a sign of the passing of time.

The sun god Helios is regarded as the bringer of sight, as the healer of the blind.

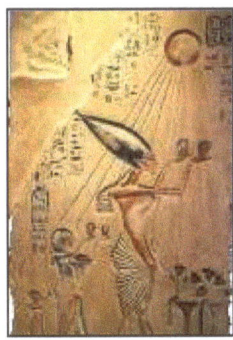
The ancient Egyptian depictions show the king and Pharaoh Akhenaton with his family sitting under the rays of the sun, receiving life's information.

Aesculapius, the god of medicine, was a son of the light god Phoebus Apollo, the "shining one". Already in Apollos' sanatoriums the doctors exposed their patients to the sun.

The first written news about the effects of light can be found at the "Father of History", Herodotus (490 BC). He noticed that the Egyptians dried meat, small poultry and fish in the sun. He could also convince himself that the skulls of the Egyptians were harder than those of the Persians when exposed to the sun. (2) Egyptians lived outside under the sun, while Persians were known as stay-at-homes.

Hippocrates, the Príncipes medicinae, born 460 BC, noticed that the inhabitants of sunny regions had a more cheerful character. People in northern climates tend to be sadder, especially in winter. Thus, for the first time, he established a connection to the currently recognized disease of seasonal depression (SAD).

The Greek-Roman physician Galen (ca. 150 BC) recommended that patients with skin diseases stay in the south, where the sun's rays are stronger.

Already the doctors of the Roman Empire used sunlight treatment for certain indications such as general weakness, obesity and arthritis.

"Get out of my sun," Diogenes said to Alexander the Great. The enjoyment of the sun was more important to him than anything else.

"Where the sun shines, the doctor does not come", a German proverb clearly states.

A German colloquial phrase describes particularly beautiful weather: "that is weather to father heroes".

An ancient Roman tradition of sunbathing after a meal is still being held today in the Italian Alpine valleys. So it is the Ticino custom to go out to the sun after a meal: "prendere il sole".

In the Middle Ages, the spreading Christian faith prohibited both sunbathing and sunlight applications. All-time chaste body covering was required.

During the industrial revolution in northern Europe in the 17th/18th century, the link between sunlight and human health became evident. People moved from the countryside to the city to work in the factories. The miserable living conditions of the industrial workers, especially their children, who were forced to work in dark factory halls and mines even in their earliest years, led to a massive lack of sunshine and vitamin D respectively. Severe bone deformities such as rickets were the result.
It was not until the end of the 19th century that people began to understand the connection between sun exposure and malnutrition and vitamin D synthesis.
In colonial times English doctors observed that patients with psoriasis had fewer relapses in sunny India than in their homeland

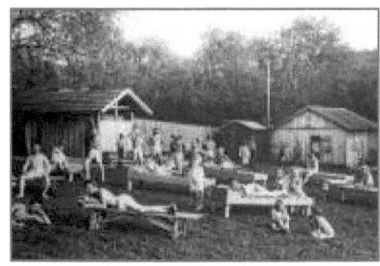

Sunbathing really came into fashion around 1900. The Zurich city clerk noted in the 1907 minutes of the city council: "The success of the many air and sun baths that are taking place everywhere is a striking proof that we are dealing here with a quite popular movement".

"Soon the sun-tanned complexion was transformed from a stigma of agricultural workers and seafarers into a coveted code. Sun tan stood for sportiness and naturalness, for health, success and sexual attractiveness, for feminine beauty and youthfulness and for male performance and immunity," writes the Zurich historian Niklaus Ingold in his book *Lichtduschen*. (3)

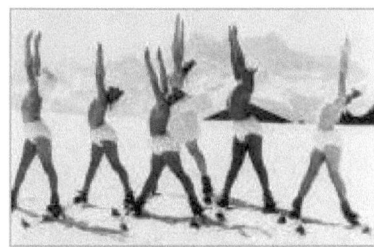

Oskar Bernhard opened the first clinic of heliotherapy in Switzerland in 1895. Auguste Rollier specialized in heliotherapies for tuberculosis patients at his Swiss clinic in Leysin. The infectious disease caused by bacteria was a major and unsolved problem until well after the Second World War.

However, Rollier supplemented therapeutic sunbathing with fitness and work. Almost naked, he let his patients exercise in the open air. And that had an effect. Sunlight stimulates the formation of vitamin D, which in turn strengthens the immune system.

The British physician Sir Edward Mellanby received the Nobel Prize in Chemistry in 1928 for the discovery of vitamin D. The production of vitamin D marked the beginning of a new era in medicine. Industry also began producing products enriched with vitamin D.

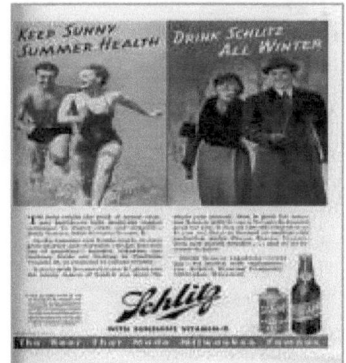

In 1936, the large brewery in Milwaukee brewed a winter beer enriched with vitamin D with the slogan: "Drink Schlitz all winter - and keep your sunny summer health" and "Schlitz - with sunshine Vitamin D".
A variety of vitamin D-enriched products entered the market.

The doctors of that time registered about 183 different diseases associated with a lack of sun rays or vitamin D. These include diabetes type 1, high blood pressure, breast cancer, gingivitis, influenza, rickets, pregnancy risks, sickle cell anemia, gestational diabetes, multiple sclerosis, depression, asthma, fibromyalgia, obesity, congestive heart failure, Parkinson's disease, dementia, cystic fibrosis, Raynaud's syndrome, hip fractures, aging, prostate cancer, Crohn's disease, allergies, obesity and many more.

Then came a disastrous turnaround. With the discovery of antibiotics in 1941, these natural, well-tried healing methods were being replaced.

In the following 50 years, medicine and the world of bacteria developed further. Bacteria became smarter, recognized the mechanism of antibiotics and were no longer so easily impressed by this 'wonder weapon'. The first antibiotic resistances frightened patients and doctors. A partial return to sunlight began. The scientists used this break from the antibiotic realm to develop new methods of light therapy in the form of UV technologies - with excellent results.

What is in the sun that allows plants to grow, attracts bees, makes hearts happy, heals wounds, takes away the sting of aging and illuminates the rooms?

Part 1
The Sun – the Bridge into the Invisible

Spring. The first rays of the sun brighten our day, the heart beats effort-lessly, and the heaviness of winter has disappeared. Spring is a happy time. Hormonal balance also adapts to the brighter frequency. Love, light, buds, green, blossoms, birdsong and spring-cleaning - we wake up from winter density, coming out of low sun intensity.

With the naked eye we see the sun as a huge fireball. For thousands of years researchers, philosophers and above all astronomers have been studying this star of the outer third of the Milky Way. With a diameter of 1.4 million kilometers, it is said to be 149.6 million kilometers away from Earth. A ray of light from the sun to the earth takes about 8 minutes to the earth. One square meter of sun shines brighter than 1 million light bulbs.

Sunlight is part of electromagnetic radiation comprised of Infrared, visible and ultraviolet light are among others. On Earth, sunlight is filtered through the Earth's atmosphere and is perceived as daylight as soon as the Sun is above the horizon.

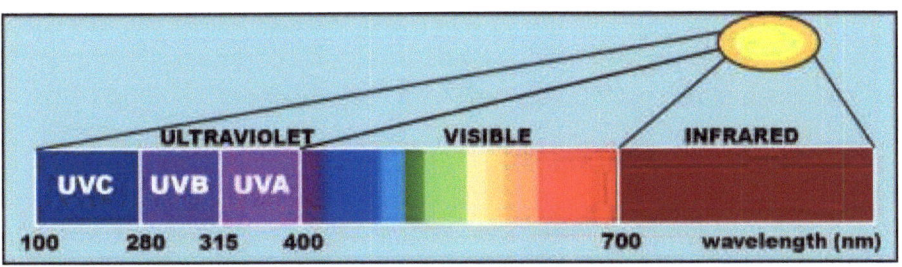

Only 5% of the sun's rays that hit the earth are UV rays. Two types of UV rays reach the Earth's surface, UVA and UVB.

UVC rays of 100 to 280 nm are the shortest wavelengths of ultraviolet light. These are blocked by the ozone layer. UVC light damages the human body.

UVB rays, 280 to 315 nm, are strongly absorbed by the earth's atmosphere. Its range is a very narrow segment of the entire ultraviolet spectrum. But it is precisely these rays that are important for vitamin D synthesis in humans and animals.

UVA rays, 315 to 400 nm, make up 95% of the ultraviolet rays that reach the earth's surface. UVA radiation is not absorbed so efficiently so it penetrates deep into the dermis and can cause skin damage.

UVA-Radiation 315 bis 400 nm	UVB-Radiation 280 bis 314 nm
Direct tan lasts only hours	Delayed, long lasting tan
No skin protection through pigmentation	Good skin protection through pigmentation
Causes skin aging	Vitamin D production - DNA specific
Produces many free radicals	Minimal production of free radicals

Only UVB radiation is responsible for vitamin D production by the sun. Thus equaling 1 - 5 % of the total UV radiation of the sun.

On the one hand, the sun is a mediator of life and yet it destroys life on the other. We measure the sun by its effect. The sun brings the day the brightness and its disappearance leads to night's darkness. Only quantum physics has the power to grant us a deeper understanding of the sun.

Quantum physics – the bridge to invisibility

While classical physics deals with matter, visible and measurable facts, quantum physics is the connecting element between biology and physics, the bridge between material and non-material parts of a living organism. This is precisely the key to understanding living systems: the alteration between the material and the non-material, between the dividable and the undividable.

> Nikola Tesla said:
> "The day science will begin to study non-physical phenomena, it will make greater progress in a decade than in all the preceding centuries of its existence.

Quantum physics deals with the undividable. The undividable, the smallest quantum of sunlight is a photon.

The Photon – the smallest light quantum

As interaction or force carrier, the photon belongs to the bosons and thus to the elementary particles.
In quantum mechanics and quantum field theory, these are particles that mediate an interaction between two systems by being emitted by one system and absorbed by the other.

- A photon is the smallest light quanta.
- A photon is a dimensionless and chargeless quantum unit of space with an oscillating electromagnetic field.
- A photon is carrier and transmitter of information.
- A photon creates a coherent field.
- A photon has zero rest mass and moves at the speed of light or faster within a vacuum.

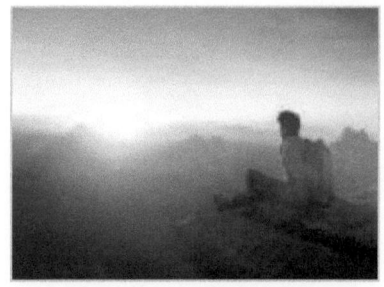

Light is a fascinating mystery that is present everywhere. Each living cell emits more than 100,000 light pulses per second. This emission of light does not end until death. Photons in a living, organic system - such as humans, animals, plants and earth - are biophotons.

They possess all the properties of photons - but they are more versatile.

"At the quantum level, we humans consist of a highly coherent field of photons capable of controlling all bodily processes." (4) For about one billion metabolic processes per second in the body, just as many billion processes of impulses and information exchange in the body. They are continuously essential for survival. Photons regulate these processes. They trigger an action and transmit certain information. We recognize and measure them only by their effect. That's why we call them "change effect particles". They come from another frequency level, set an impulse and thus trigger an action.

The body has about 22 organs, 246 bones, 650 muscles and 143 joints.
Every minute 600 million cells die and new cells are being built. There is no interruption in communication.
Each of the 700 billion cells receives several 1,000 action messages per second. All processes are coordinated at the speed of light or even faster.

Prof. Dr. Popp, the world-renowned biophoton researcher, said: "The way in which information and energy are transmitted by photons shows us that we are held together in our core by nothing other than light quanta. (5)

Based on today's overall biophoton research:

Biophotons - in the human system

- Biophotons are photons in a living organic system.
- Biophotons are carriers and transmitters of information and triggers of actions.
- Biophotons are responsible for communication in all life, from individual cells to entire organisms - also for cell division and cell-to-cell communication.
- Communication takes place at the speed of light.
- Biophotons penetrate cell layers without loss.
- Biophotons create a coherent living field of order.
- DNA is a biophoton memory bank.
- Blu Room produces biophoton equilibrium, density or condensation.

All this happens with the highest precision, thanks to the coherence of the light.

Coherence – order by light

Every living substance, every healthy, organic cell of plants, humans and animals emit a weak, but highly ordered, uniform, i.e. coherent, phase-stable light. The word coherence means order.

"Ordered means that the ability exists to carry out an interaction in which each part can communicate with each other," Dr. Popp is convinced. (5)

Coherence theory speaks of a coherent light connection between the genetic control center, the DNA, and all other cell components in the cell.

Homeopathy and acupuncture are based on the presence of coherent and structured light.

Prof. Fritz Albert Popp sees a coherent biophoton field as an expression of optimal cell health. The energy field enables the optimal communication of its components among each other as well as the communication of the organ with the information field of the whole organism. The more coherent the energy field, the more effectively the organ is connected to its information field.

A coherence field builds up in water, for example, when all water molecules oscillate in the same rhythm. In this equal swinging structure, a collision of the individual molecules can be avoided and the individual molecule consumes less energy.

However, if the coherence is weaker, the communication between the organ and its information field is disturbed. This can lead to disorder and health problems.

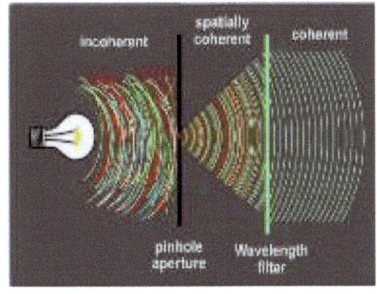

Scientists at Ryerson University in Canada use this image to clearly show how a chaotic field changes into an ordered field under the influence of light. (6)

Coherent states or the state of the biophoton field are an indicator of the extent to which a system oscillates in harmony with its environment. The aim is to maintain or restore the biological regulatory capacity of the organs and the entire body.

The abundance of biophotons is neutral and gives us the energy for both - life decreasing and life creating.

Negative influences are e.g. psychological and physical stress, environmental toxins, the type of nutrition, contaminated foods, inflammations, bacteria and viruses and personal thought patterns. They disturb the harmony of the frequencies of the electromagnetic field, i.e. the coherence in our body.

For the coherence of a field, both the concentration, i.e. the quantity as well as the quality of the photons is of decisive importance.

Coherence - order through light

- Coherent light waves are light waves of the same wavelength and phase.
- Coherence describes the vitality and energy state of the system.
- Coherence is absolute order, pressure-free state and communication.
- Photons have long coherence times (order times).
- A coherent state builds the bridge between autonomous and somatic (individual) systems.
- Blu Room UVB light generates coherence.

A short excursion into food:
The higher the light storage capacity of the food, the better the integration of irradiated light into the human/plant/animal life network. The more intensive the order of light storage, the higher the biological quality. So it is not vitamins and nutrient content that determine the liveliness of food, but the order of light storage and coherence.

Close the door. No one is allowed to look in! The room of a Teenager. The curtains are closed. From the parent's point of view there is pure chaos, pure disorder, nothing is going on. The teenager doesn't see it so narrowly. Everything he doesn't want to clean up ends up in his room. Is that a disease? No, it's just disorder. Often only an external impulse for example the first love is enough to bring light, order and happiness into this room. The cleaning up begins. Open the window, bring in light. Useless items are thrown out, socks are tidily arranged next to underwear, and even school documents are neatly labelled. Even the curtains smell of freshness and freedom. The sun covers the room in soft light.

It is the same in our body. When ballast accumulates in the cell, communication no longer works flawlessly. Lack of light leads to disorder. Disorder can turn into order through light.

Medicine gives the disorder a name that matches the locality. Diabetes or renal carcinoma. Fear already resonates as a serious additional disorder factor.

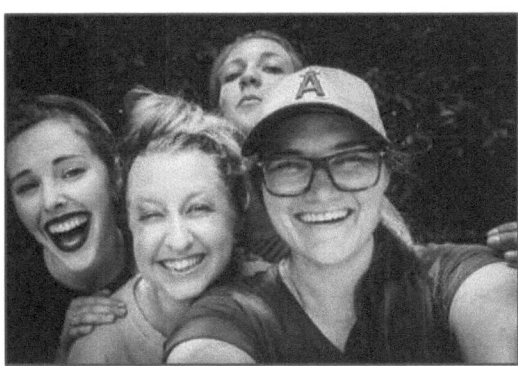

Every person is unique, brilliant, and individual. That's a good thing. This makes everyone valuable and brings us closer to our greater mission. Every human being has his own life code or life plan. This code is located in the DNA.

In 1899 Nikola Tesla said: Everything that is is light.

DNA – the photon controlled master plan

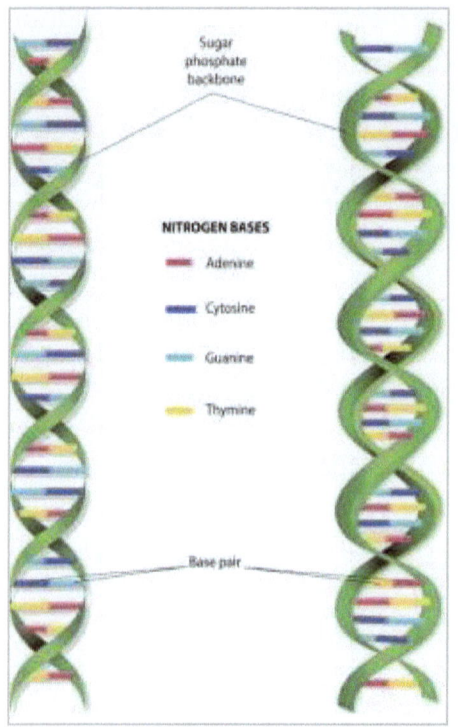

From a biological point of view, every cell of our body, protected by the nucleus, contains an organic macromolecule, the DNA. It is the carrier of the genetic code. In this macromolecule all information of the development, the function and the individuality of the living being are generally and individually coded. This is the blueprint with which we are born.

Roughly speaking, the DNA molecule is like a huge zipper. Stretched out, a DNA molecule would have a length of almost two meters. We would not be able to see it with our naked eyes because it would only be about seven millionths of a centimeter thick.

In order to accommodate something so gigantic in every human cell nucleus, "the DNA simply rolls itself into a tightly rolled ball.
The double strand first winds like a spiral spring or double helix. This then rotates and turns until it fits into a space of only about one billionth of a cubic centimeter." (7)

28

DNA is a quantum wave

Until now, science has assumed that DNA is merely a macromolecule. In 2017, Lance Shuttler published new scientific experiments. He confirms that "DNA originates from a quantum wave and not as a molecule". He writes: "The photons shoot back and forth rhythmically in the DNA at the speed of light, and are stored until they are needed." (8)

Western scientists have long assumed that only a maximum of 10-20% of this DNA is important for human life. Russian scientists were the first to introduce a much larger dimension of DNA. They discovered that an enormous part of the DNA molecule serves communication and information purposes, i.e. is a huge control apparatus. "Every strand of DNA," says Lance Shuttler, "goes hand in hand with a strand of light."

The DNA acts as a rod antenna and simultaneously as a ring antenna.

DNA is an ideal electromagnetic antenna.
- One part is elongated and thus a rod antenna, which can absorb electrical impulses very well.
- At the same time, seen from above, it is ring-shaped and therefore a very good magnetic antenna. (7)

In this way, our DNA can absorb electromagnetic radiation, i.e. light from the environment. The molecule vibrates due to the activity of the photons, thus making it possible for the DNA to store energy.

This interaction of the antennas makes the DNA an ideal resonator for visible sunlight.

DNA - the photon controlled master plan

- DNA is the carrier of genetic information, therefore it is the physical basis of all genes.
- Every disease is a light metabolic disorder.
- DNA is a photon storage and information transmitter.
- DNA contains all information from the genotype and phenotype.
- In the DNA all information for the development, the function and the individuality of each living being is stored in a coded form. These are the genes or hereditary predispositions.

After fertilization different cells form. But all cells know that they belong in a human system - and not, for example, in a mouse system. In order for a cell to know what it should look like and what function it plays in the organism, each cell has all this information in coded form in the genes working in the cell nucleus, in the DNA. Put simply, the DNA is the code, construction plan or blueprint.

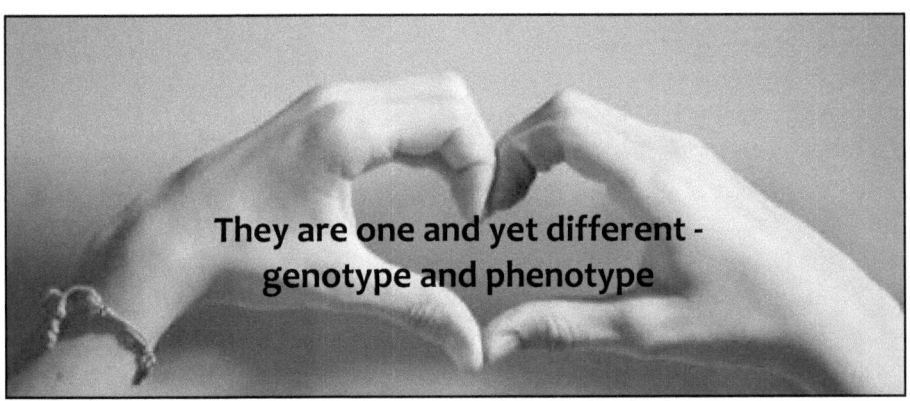

They are one and yet different - genotype and phenotype

Looking at the reproductive process, it is easier for us to understand the two types. The very first cell, also called stem cell, already contains a perfect set of DNA, the geno- and the phenotype.

Genotype
The cell knows according to its blueprint: I will be a human being. Every person on this planet has a head, a torso, two arms, two legs, certain organs and the functional scheme of an optimally healthy person. This is the genotype part, the optimal, unchangeable life matrix.
Medicine speaks of an autonomous basic plan which is the same for all people, the genotype. This does not change during the lifetime of an organism.

Phenotype
At the same time, the first omnipotent stem cell knows: this human cell be a girl, brown hair, dark eyes, and all individual aspects. This individual information comes from the genetic pool of the father and the mother. This is the pheno-component of DNA.

Phenotype is a description of the actual physical characteristics. This includes straightforward visible characteristics like height and eye color, but also overall health, disease history, and even behavior and general disposition. Does one gain weight easily? Is the person anxious or calm? Does he like cats? These are all the ways in which one presents himself to the world, and as such are considered phenotypes.

Most phenotypes are influenced by both the genotype and by the unique circumstances in which one has lived his life, including everything that has ever happened to him. (9)

This phenotype corresponds to the individual aspect of DNA, like a matrix. This DNA is changeable.

> Did grandmother starve to death on the run, has grandfather been a successful businessman, the mother a profound Christian, the great-grandson a famous composer, the great-uncle a math genius, the great-great-grandfather loved a gypsy... all this is a huge pool of hereditary traits from which the phenotype of the new DNA is formed.

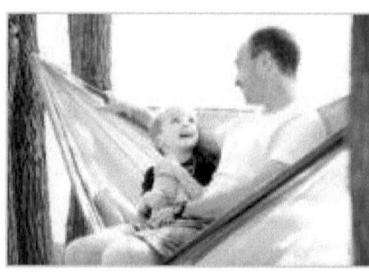

When the child grows up, we see "typically great-uncle Albert, the math genius; the artistic talent is from great-uncle Chuck; the hand for business he has from grandmother Lina, the unsteady life can only come from the gypsy blood, and the crooked toes are from grandfather Brian".

The genotype knows only one program: a life of light and pure coherence.

The phenotype in its individuality brings chances and challenges. This is the beauty and attraction of life, and calls for change, growth and constructive togetherness. A persistence in old life programs binds or blocks light. Due to the lack of light, the pheno system tends to incoherence and disorder.

Prof. Dr. Popp says that every disease has at the root a disturbance of the light metabolism, or lack of light. (5)

Green leaf – red blood– blue light

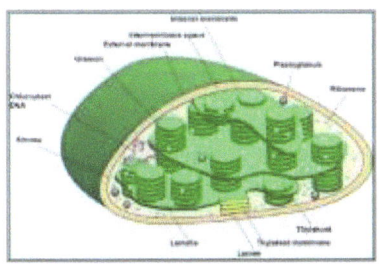

One of the most effective light-submitting substances on our planet is chlorophyll. Chlorophyll is the color pigment that gives plants their green color and enables them to photosynthesize. An ingenious biophysicist at the University of Michigan Jennifer Ogilvie discovered the secret behind chlorophyll in March 2018. (10) Her scientific team depicted the moment when a photon triggered the first steps of photosynthesis for energy conversion.

In photosynthesis, light hits the chlorophyll, which is embedded in so-called light-collecting antenna complexes. These are small, spherical structures, the chloroplasts.

In the chloroplasts, there are photon complexes stacked like money rolls in different "floors", in which the actual chlorophyll is stored. This gives the chloroplasts their green appearance.

The individual chlorophyll molecules are not randomly distributed in the stacks, but together form "light photon traps" together. They absorb the light of certain wavelengths and bundle the energy obtained this way via "antennas" which are stored in the membrane of the stacks.

Prof. Ogilvie says: "You can imagine it like a battery." (10)

The resulting product? Oxygen in plants and photons for the human organism.

This energy conversion takes place faster than lightning - within a few piko-seconds. Piko-seconds are a trillionth of a second, an incomprehensible short time span.

What connects the human body with chlorophyll and photosynthesis?

The chemical similarity between the red blood pigment hemoglobin and chlorophyll is striking.

Chlorophyll and the hemoglobin in the red blood cells are twins in their chemical structure. The only difference is that the central element in chlorophyll is magnesium and in hemoglobin the molecule is iron.

The iron atom in hemoglobin binds oxygen and thus ensures oxygen transport in the body. Magnesium is responsible for the ability to absorb sunlight.

Photons give the chlorophyll in the plant the color green.

Photons give the hemoglobin in the blood the color red.

Sun generating Chlorophyll

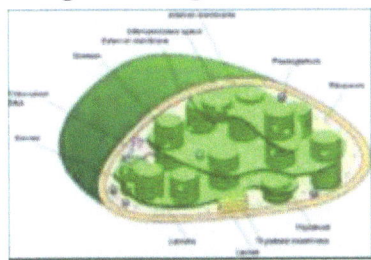

Sun generating Vitamin D

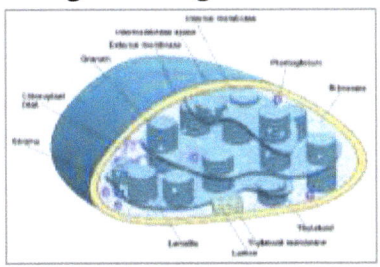

Chlorophyll in the plant
Chlorophyll is the Vitamin D of the plant,
It is a photon storage
Energy and information,
DNA frequency-specific,
It is coherent,

Vitamin D in humans
formed from fat-soluble cholesterol.
It is a photon storage,
Energy and information,
Vitamin D3 is the only vitamin that
the body makes by itself
DNA frequency specific, coherent.

Effect of chlorophyll in the human organism
- can be blood cleansing and hematopoietic,
- can balance metabolism of acid and bases,
- may be anticarcinogenic,
- may have an antibacterial effect,
- may regulate healthy bacterial growth,
- may have an antioxidant effect, bind free radicals,
- may have a regenerative effect on radiation damage.

Effect of Vitamin D in the human organism
- Vitamin D controls more than 3,000 genes.
- Vitamin D has an effect on DNA,
- on the mineral metabolism,
- Effects on the immune system, heart and circulation.
- Effects on nerves and brain
- Effects on metabolism and epigenetics
- Viability and duration
- Thoughts, inner stability, self-confidence
- Mental and spiritual abilities
- Vitamin D can switch genes on and off

PART 2
Vitamin D – the Hidden Potential

Only UVB radiation is responsible for the vitamin D production by the sun. Thus 1 - 5 % of the total UV radiation of the sun.

Vitamin D production by the sun is individual and depends on:
- Latitude and season (sun intensity)
- skin pigmentation
- altitude
- ozone layer
- reflection on the earth's surface, clouds
- air pollution
- age, sex, weight, skin type, health situation

Effect of Vitamin D in the human organism

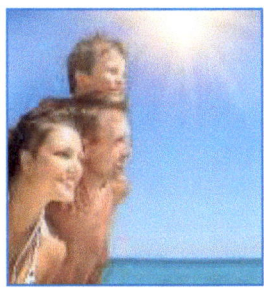

Vitamin D controls more than 3,000 genes and thus has a huge influence on the function of cells, organs and entire systems. The effects of vitamin D can be seen throughout the body and in the psyche.

Vitamin D receptor sites – docking stations
Through sunlight our skin forms 25-OH-Calcidiol, the inactive form of vitamin D. From this, the active form 1,25-OH-Calcitriol is built in the kidney. This then is responsible for the various vitamin D effects in the cell. To enter the cell, calcitriol first couples to a vitamin D receptor (VDR). This receptor is thus activated and triggers numerous other processes and regulatory mechanisms, including the control of our DNA.

Two physicians at Indira Gandhi Open University, Ahmedabad, India, describe in detail the activities of the vitamin D receptor (VDR) as a binding protein. The receptor binds vitamin D to "genes and regulates the synthesis of numerous proteins, enzymes and neurotransmitters, which in turn control and influence numerous physical processes". (11) The vitamin D receptor also significantly influences genes associated with cancer and autoimmune diseases. (12)

Vitamin D receptors are found throughout the body on almost every single one of the 700 billion cells, from sperm to mitochondria. (13)

Here are some examples:
- Eyes (14)
- Pancreas (15)
- Breasttissue (16)
- Fatty tissue (11)
- Brain (13)
- Immune system (17)
- Skin (18) and muscle (19)
- Bones (20)
- Liver (21) and kidney (11)
- Thyroid and gonads (22)
- Nervous system (23)
- Prostate (24)
- DNA (25)

The Bridge from being sick to being healthy

Man consists of body, soul and spirit. He strives by nature for unity, health and healing. Health is individual and is defined by a state that reflects the harmony and functionality of the whole person.
If we understand the following basic principle of being healthy and not being healthy, then it is child's play to recognize the immeasurable effect of vitamin D and Blu Room. The "bridge" from the optimal, coherent life matrix to the individually shaped incoherent matrix becomes evident.

As we already discovered with the division of the DNA matrix into two intertwined parts, all body systems act according to a vital double matrix. Basically, we are born with all autonomous systems in optimal order. The optimal, unchangeable life matrix determines the individual, changeable matrix in our lives. Individual events, genetic patterns, experiences in wars, famines, education, environment, nutrition, social awareness and one's own thinking influence this individual aspect. When we are stressed, the adrenal gland reacts by emitting stress hormones. These in turn disturb the orderly flow within the system. Health disturbances build up over a long period of time.

> A photon is the smallest light quantum.
>
> Biophotons penetrate cell layers without loss.
>
> Biophotons build a coherent living field of order.

The system is in disorder due to a lack of light. Vitamin D is like a photon capsule. Where it is present, it ensures order. The cell is stimulated by photons to order, repair and spur on to correct structure.

Many double-blind, placebo-controlled studies worldwide have identified a severe vitamin D deficiency as one of the causes of many diseases.

This graph from 2013 gives us a good overview. It shows the relationship between vitamin D levels and diseases - Grassroots Health June 2013 (16)

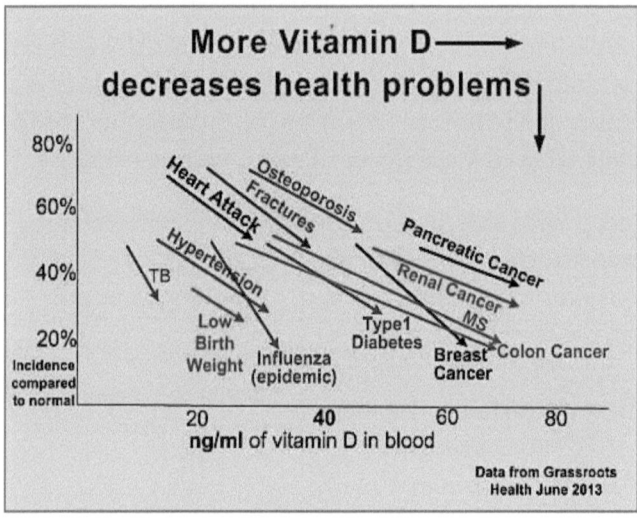

pancreatic cancer
breast cancer
fractures
low birth weight
gestosis
flu epidemic
kidney cancer,
intestinal cancer
osteoporosis,
diabetes type 1
multiple sclerosis
high blood pressure
stroke, heart attack
tuberculosis, asthma
high blood pressure

Source: www.grassrootshealth.net

Immune system and photon carrier vitamin D

The immune system functions like a mobile task force and consists of a network of cells, tissues and organs. It controls the body's own processes and protects the body against pathogens in their interaction with the environment.

> *The immune system operates analogously to the DNA types with its autonomous as well as its individual genetic matrix. Medicine speaks of*
> - *the autonomic, innate immune system and the*
> - *adaptive immune system.*

We are born with all the abilities of the autonomous immune system. The acquired, specialized immune defense only develops in the course of the individual's life and reacts to personal experiences such as critical life events, feelings and actions.
Both systems are closely interlocked in their mode of operation and nevertheless take on different tasks.
It is the individual aspects of a person (phenotype) that lead to disturbances in the immune system, light deficiency and incoherence. If there is no order, the light or photon carrier is missing in the form of vitamin D in the body.

Some diseases show this clearly. (See also the master work: *Blu Room - Experience the future* (1)

Asthma attacks and vitamin D

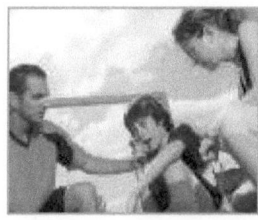

Asthma is a very common disease. It affects about 300 million people worldwide. Typical symptoms are a whistling sound, shortness of breath, chest tightness and cough. The enormous influence of vitamin D works in the innate and acquired immune system.

Queen Mary University of London published a study in 2016. The leading professor, Adrian Martineau of the Asthma UK Center for Applied Research could clearly prove that "an oral vitamin D intake in addition to standard asthma drugs significantly reduced severe asthma attacks". (26)

Protection against influenza with vitamin D – for all ages

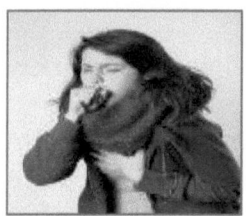

The annual flu season usually begins with the decrease in sun intensity. In the low light months, people spend more of their time indoors. Less sunlight means less vitamin D. Not the virus causes a flu, but an immune system weakened by a strong vitamin D deficiency.

Vitamin D controls the innate immune defense and is vital for well-being.

A study published in the year 2006 shows that 90% of the participants with sufficient vitamin D intake remained spared of the flu. (27) 30% of participants with low vitamin D levels suffered from a cold. (28)

Sufficient vitamin D levels can improve the protection of older people from influenza diseases after influenza vaccination. (29)

The Japanese researchers concluded that "additional vitamin D intake reduces the risk of influenza infection more effectively than vaccines or antiviral drugs". The result was published in the *American Journal of Clinical Nutrition* in 2010. (30)

Neurodermatitis and vitamin D and UVB

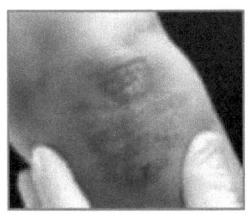 Cholecalciferol, known as vitamin D3, influences many reactions in the human body. The skin can be very sensitive to vitamin D deficiency and can respond with eczema such as neurodermatitis or atopic dermatosis. The symptoms often worsen in winter.

"A healthy skin produces antimicrobial peptides as a defense against viruses and bacteria. In patients with inflammatory skin diseases such as psoriasis or neurodermatitis, the natural balance of these peptides is disturbed," says private lecturer Dr. Jürgen Schauber at the Dermatological Clinic of the University Hospital Munich. (31) Together with Finnish colleagues he concluded: "If the skin of psoriasis and neurodermatitis patients is irradiated with ultraviolet light, low vitamin D levels are corrected". Vitamin D in turn alters the activity of cathelicidin and presumably other antimicrobial peptides. (32)

Scleroderma, psoriasis in combination with vitamin D and UVB

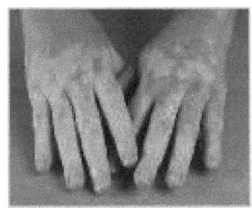 Psoriasis is a skin disease characterized by inflammation and scaling of the skin. Psoriasis can also affect joints and nails. (Rheumatoid arthritis). After the discovery of ultraviolet radiation in 1896, Dr. Niels Ryberg Finsen began to treat all types of skin diseases with UV radiation. The radiation kills pathogenic microorganisms. At the same time, the skin produces vitamin D. Thus the immunity in the human body increases. "Complete cures were reported in 80% of cases." (33) Finsen was awarded the Nobel Prize in 1903 for his outstanding achievements.

In a 1986 study, patients with psoriasis received both an oral dose of vitamin D and a direct treatment of the affected areas with vitamin D-containing oil. Improvements were observed in 76% of patients at the end of the study after eight weeks. (33)
Similar study results in the field of immune system and vitamin D were found for: Infectious diseases of all types, autoimmune diseases, allergies and congenital or acquired immunodeficiency. (34)

Radioactive damage drastically reduced by vitamin D and UVB

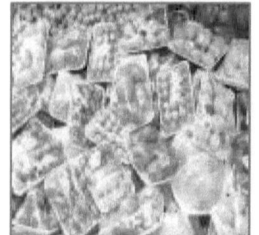

In 2010, the Saarland group of Prof. W. Tilgen and Jörg Reichrath from the University of Homburg / Saar confirmed the protection of skin cells by calcitriol in a cell experiment. This protects the skin cells from damage caused by ionizing radiation. (35)

During the atomic bomb tests in the South Pacific (Bikini Atoll), the people living there were more exposed to radiation than the observing soldiers on the ships from the USA and Great Britain. However, leukemia developed as a result of radiation overdose in the soldiers. People in the South Seas rarely got this type of cancer. (36)

Exposure to bisphenol A (BPA) and other endocrine-disrupting chemicals may alter the active form of vitamin D in body

In September 2016, the Endocrine Society, based in Washington, D.C., USA, published for the first time in its *Journal of Clinical Endocrinology & Metabolism* a study on the effects of bisphenol A (BPA) and other endocrine-disrupting chemicals, also known as phthalates.

These substances have shown an ability to reduce vitamin D levels in the blood. (37)

BPA could even be found in fresh greenhouse fruit and drinking water. Most BPA is absorbed from food, especially through plastics in drinking bottles, storage cans, foil packaging, body care products, children's products and medical tubing.

More than 1,300 studies revealed health problems, including infertility, obesity, diabetes, neurological problems and hormone-related cancers. "Almost every person on the planet is exposed to BPA and a different class of endocrine disrupting chemicals. This can lead to widespread public health effects by reducing vitamin D," says leading author Lauren Johns, MPH, a PhD student at the University Of Michigan School Of Public Health in Ann Arbor, MI. (38)

Nervous system and the photon carrier vitamin D

Our body is a complex and sensitive information community with the nervous system acting as a highly specialized network. A nerve cell or neuron is a cell specialized in conduction and transmission of stimulation. Its task is the communication and processing of signals between cells, organs and body parts. The nervous system allows us to perceive, understand and react to the world around us.

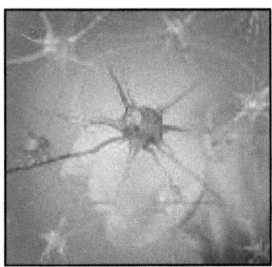

For thousands of years man has reacted to an acute threat according to two original reactions: Fight or flight. The human being must adapt as quickly as possible to a suddenly occurring dangerous situation.

The sympathetic nervous system regulates the stress reaction of the body and is activated during increased physical and psychological stress. The sympathetic nervous system regulates energy storage and digestion. It steers the heart to a slower frequency and stimulates blood circulation in the periphery and intestines by means of vasodilatation. Ultimately, an interaction between individual genetic factors and the environment is omnipresent.

All disturbances of the nervous system derive from the individual aspects of the systems and are therefore caused independently. Any disturbance in the nervous system is a disturbance of the optimal order. A lack of light causes this.

The nervous system operates analogously to the DNA types with its autonomous matrix as well as its individual genetic matrix. Medicine speaks of:
- *Autonomic, unchangeable nervous system and the*
- *Somatic or vegetative, variable nervous system.*

Effect of vitamin D as a photon carrier in the nervous system

Prevention of oxidative damage to nerve tissue and increases glutathione levels. (39)

- Support of detoxification and correct formation and maintenance of neuronal connections.
- Controlling the cell cycle of nerve cells and neuroplasticity. (40)
- Influence on the synthesis of neurotransmitters and supports cell-to-cell communication.
- Controlling the formation of important antioxidants and influences brain detoxification.
- Regulation the expression of over 2,000 genes. (41)
- Support of intracellular Calcium homeostasis,
- Stimulation. (40)
- Vitamin D repairs the myelin sheath. Remyelination is the restoration of the myelin sheath of nerve fibers after damage.

Depression and vitamin D

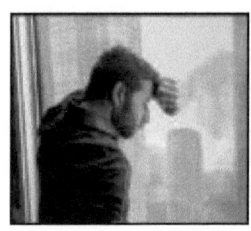

Today, depression is one of the most frequent and at the same time most serious mental illness. Many possible causes such as genetic predisposition, neuro-biological disorders, certain development and personality factors, stressful life events, medication, and toxins such as glysophate and health problems lead to depression.

Depressed people often have an extremely low vitamin D level. (42) The link between vitamin D levels and depression was confirmed by researchers from the Department of Psychiatry and Behavioral Neuroscience at St. Joseph's Hospital in Hamilton, Ontario province, Canada. (196)

The more impressive the vitamin D deficiency is, the more severe are the symptoms of depression. (43)

Mood swings during pregnancy and vitamin D

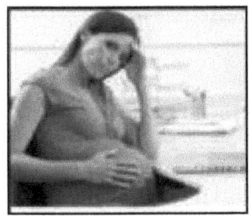

Severe mood swings during pregnancy and after childbirth are common. About twelve percent of expectant mothers develop a manifest depression. Half of the women who suffer from severe depression during pregnancy slip into postpartum depression.

Iranian physicians investigated the correlation between low serum Vitamin D levels and prenatal depression. The study, published in 2016, showed that "a daily intake of 2,000 I.E. vitamin D3 during late pregnancy effectively prevented childbed depression". (44)

Autism and vitamin D

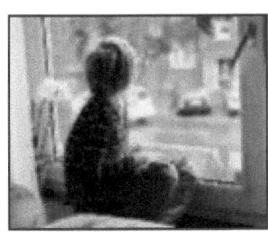

Autism, one variant of which is Asperger's syndrome, is one of the most profound developmental disorders. Complex disturbances of the central nervous system are evident - especially in the area of processing perception.

Vitamin D plays an important role in neuronal development and gene regulation. More than 3,000 genes contain Vitamin D receptors.

A randomized and controlled double-blind study with 109 autistic children aged between three and ten years helped clarify the relationship between autism and vitamin D deficiency in 2016. The physicians involved in the study concluded: "Children with vitamin D supplementation developed higher cognitive awareness and significantly better social maturity than children in the placebo group. (45)

Morbus Parkinson and vitamin D

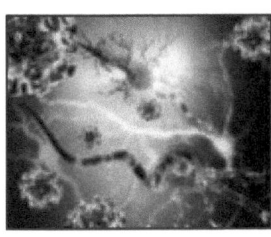

Parkinson's disease is a slowly progressive degeneration of the nervous system. It is triggered by the death of cells in an area of the midbrain, the substantia nigra. The main symptoms are muscle tremors, slower movements and/or muscle stiffness.

A 2016 study showed lower vitamin D levels in Parkinson's patients compared to healthy individuals of the same age (46) Scientists found the largest amount of vitamin D receptors in the substantia nigra, the dopamine-rich region. They suggest that this explains the neuroprotective role of vitamin D in several brain disorders, including Parkinson's disease and Alzheimer's disease. (47)

Dr. Nicolai Worms clarifies in his book *Heilkraft Vitamin D*: "Such degenerative diseases always have several causes. A vitamin D deficiency alone cannot be the cause. Rather vitamin D apparently is a cofactor, a co-responsible factor in the development of the underlying disorder". (48)

Morbus Alzheimer, dementia and vitamin D

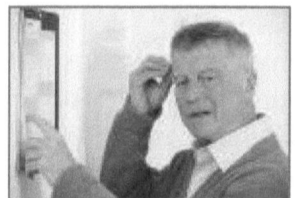

Dementia is a general term for an acquired impairment of mental performance that restricts memory, language, orientation, social behavior and judgment.

In an article published in 2014, Spiegel writes: "The less vitamin D older people have in their blood, the more likely they are to develop dementia. A recent study from the USA shows this connection. In Germany, about 60 percent of older people are affected by vitamin D deficiency". (49)

Epileptic seizures and vitamin D

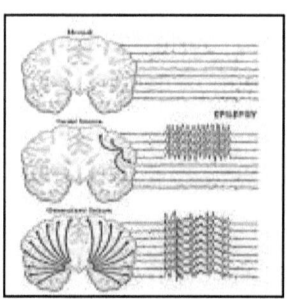

An epileptic seizure is a spasm-like functional disorder of the brain caused by a simultaneous excessive discharge of nerve cells (neurons). Hungarian researchers at the National Institute for Medical Rehabilitation, Budapest, showed a connection between vitamin D and epilepsy. "There is consistent evidence to suggest a role of vitamin D deficiency in the pathophysiology of epilepsy." (50)

A pilot study conducted in 2012 came to the following conclusion: "We found that the number of seizures decreased significantly with vitamin

D supplementation. The average seizure was decreased by 40%. We conclude that the normalization of serum vitamin 25 (OH)-D levels has an anticonvulsant effect." (51)

Multiple Sclerosis and vitamin D

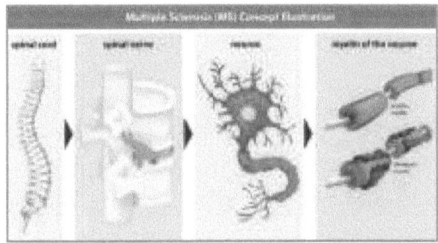

There is a very specific geographical distribution of this disease around the world. A significantly higher incidence of the malady is found in the northernmost latitudes and the southernmost latitudes. This theory was first proposed in the 1970s. (52). The starting point was the observation that the frequency of MS is associated with latitude and the UV index. Today there is numerous proof of this theory. The further away the equator is, the higher the risk of MS. Sunlight is the body's most efficient source of vitamin D - suggesting that sunlight can protect against MS. (53) Also the frequency of new illnesses and relapses increases in the dark season.

The geographical distribution of MS was particularly low in the areas rich in fish. Migration from northern to southern areas reduces the risk of multiple sclerosis. (54)

Multiple sclerosis is a chronic inflammatory disease of the central nervous system in which the marrow of the nerve process is destroyed. The myelin sheaths are ruined.

Vitamin D regulates remyelination. It promotes the development of neural stem cells into oligodendrocytes. Oligodendrocytes are the specialized cells that build the myelin sheath.

A study by the University of Maastricht in the Netherlands suggests that the "frequency, progression and severity of MS symptoms can be reduced by increasing vitamin D supplementation". (55)

The results of a study published in the *Journal of Neurology* in 2015 were not surprising.

"Low serum 25-hydroxyVitamin D (25 [OH] D) levels are associated with increased risk of MS and increased activity of the disease in early stages of MS." The study included 1,482 patients from 26 countries. The conclusions state "that adequate vitamin D levels may be an important influencing factor for MS activity not only during disease development, but also to the years thereafter. (56) "In their analysis, the researchers found a significant association between vitamin D levels and the risk of developing MS. An increase of 50 nmol /l (20ng/ml) vitamin D was associated with a 37% lower risk of MS in this study." (57)

Vitamin D stimulates growth of grey matter in the brain

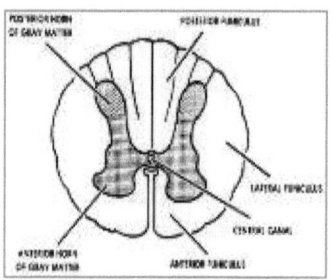

The grey substance is an important component of the central nervous system and significantly determines its functions. Especially the intelligence of the brain is associated with grey matter. However, in addition to intelligence, it controls all perceptual processes and motor functions of the human being. (58)

Source: www.indiana.edu

The grey matter is present in all parts of the central nervous system. This also applies to the brain, spinal cord and nerve pathways.

In 2015, researchers investigated the relationship between vitamin D level, grey matter volume and the extent to which vitamin D has a neuroprotective effect on MS patients.

Vitamin D council reports on this study and writes. "A vitamin D status is positively associated with the volume of grey brain matter in patients with multiple sclerosis. Grey matter is responsible for the processing of information in the brain. A reduction in the volume of grey matter in the brain reflects neuro-degeneration and disability in patients with MS". (59)

In 2016, researchers confirmed "65 patients showed an increase in grey matter volume by 7.8 ml, with an increase in vitamin D levels by 10 ng/ml. A low vitamin D status was associated with a 44% increase in new brain lesions and a relapse within one year". (60)

Comparable study results:

Polyneuropathy, progressive muscular dystrophy, fibromyalgia, paralysis, dyslexia, migraine, ADHD, scoliosis and more. See also *Blu Room - experience the future*. (34)

Metabolism and the photon carrier vitamin D

Energy production is one of the decisive tasks of metabolism. Nutrition is the key to this. The organism converts chemical substances into intermediates and end products. These biochemical processes serve to assemble and maintain the body substance as well as to generate energy for activities and to maintain bodily functions.

All metabolic organs participate in a fixed pattern. One is dependent on the other. But all are active for one goal, one lifeform and this life.

> *Like DNA, the immune and nervous systems, the metabolism also functions with its autonomous matrix, which is also individually genetically shaped. Medicine speaks of*
> - *autonomous, unchangeable metabolic system and the*
> - *psychic, modifiable metabolism system.*

The liver is the organ most active in the metabolic system. Here we see how fluently the autonomous offers the working platform to the psychic. Individual life experiences shape the psychic metabolic system.

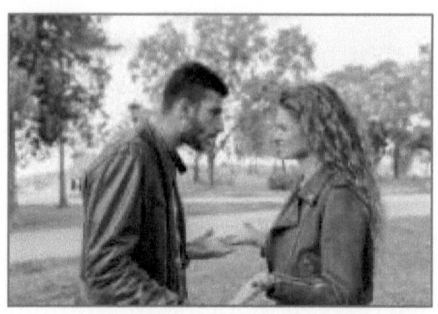

As a strategist in the body, the liver enables general structural tasks in metabolism by providing the prerequisites. If, however, unexpected external influences disrupt the smooth flow, it can be disappointed. It "gets angry". The "getting angry" or "getting upset" is a topic of liver and gall bladder. Now we are imperceptibly in the middle of a psychological metabolic process, a process that is related to our own individual perception and its reaction to it. Critical life events, financial or legal disasters, psychological and physical injuries and illnesses, separations/divorces from loved ones, job loss and mobbing, among other things, shape these processes. "The events are not decisive per se, but the subjectively felt injury, despair, helplessness or the sheer horror and fear they cause. The "viruses" are thus not the events of life itself, but the self-damaging, constricting thoughts, feelings, or actions they trigger. (61)

All disturbances of the metabolism come from the individual aspects of the systems, i.e. caused individually. Ultimately, the order of the metabolic system is disturbed. At the cellular level, a disturbed information and communication field occurs due to a lack of light or, more clearly, due to a lack of photons.

Bone health and Vitamin D and calcium

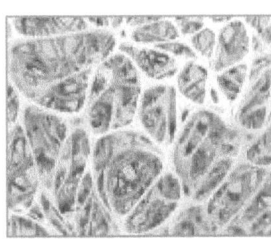 The human body contains roughly of 212 and 246 bones. The bone system is living tissue that is continuously built up and broken down. The lifespan of bone cells is between 15 and 35 years. Osteoporosis is a disorder of bone metabolism. If the bone cells lack certain building blocks, a gradual loss of bone mass occurs. "Osteoporosis affects men and women of all races, white and Asian women. The risk of women suffering from osteoporosis before the menopause is twice as high as that of men of the same age. This is the conclusion of a study by Mayo Clinic, USA (62)

Vitamin D is essential for the development and maintenance of the bone, both for its role in supporting calcium absorption from food in the gut, and for ensuring the proper renewal and mineralization of bone tissue. (63)

Vitamin D

- is essential for the correct renewal and mineralization of bone tissue.
- controls phosphate and calcium levels indirectly in the blood,
- ensures a constant blood calcium level with the parathyroid hormone,
- is responsible for the synthesis of two calcium-transporting proteins, osteocalcin and matrix GLA protein. These proteins are essential for proper bone formation.

Researchers of a three-year placebo-controlled, randomized, double-blind study investigated the effects of calcium and vitamin D supplementation on bone density in men and women over 65 years of age. After completion of the study, participants who received vitamin D and calcium showed significantly greater changes in a number of biochemical processes of bone metabolism. "Substantially positive changes were measured in the bone mineral density at the thigh neck, the spinal column and the total body. (64)

Fewer bone fractures with higher Vitamin D levels

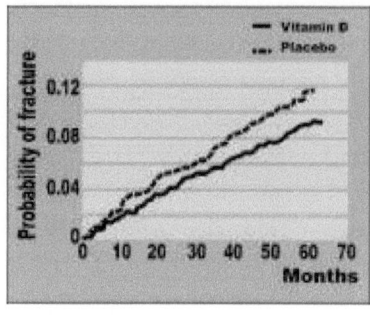

Vitamin D not only helps prevent bone loss, it also helps prevent bone fractures by strengthening muscles and nerves.

US researchers advise athletes and the elderly in particular to take vitamin D supplementation as a preventive measure against bone fractures.

Source: BMJ-Volume 326, March 1, 2003

"We recommend a serum vitamin D concentration of at least 40 ng/ml for active people with moderate or higher functional requirements to avoid fatigue fractures," explain the authors Dr. Jason R. Miller, foot and joint surgeon at the Pennsylvania Orthopedics Center in Malvern, Pennsylvania, USA. The Netherlands Journal of Medicine published study results in March 2015 with the recommendation: "For effective case and fracture prevention, an optimal value of at least 40 ng/ml is required by experts and professional associations. Values of 21 ng/ml vitamin D3 and lower are insufficient." (65)

Overweight and Vitamin D

Many people gain weight during the winter months, when the sun disappears behind grey clouds for months and vitamin D levels weaken.

The brown bear roams the countryside throughout the summer with summer sunshine intensity. The sun's vitamin D is constantly replenished and ensures an active bear life. If the intensity of the sun drops, the bear begins to prepare for hibernation triggered by the decreasing vitamin D level. He gains 70 % in body weight.

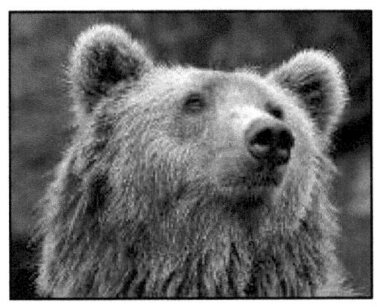

Grizzly bears gain more than 100 pounds before hibernation. Since their cells continue to react to insulin, unlike humans, they do not develop type 2 diabetes or other metabolic diseases. It is known that bear fat cells actually react to insulin depending on the season. In summer, they react more sensitively when the sun is at its highest. As soon as the bear starts to fatten, the cells become insulin-resistant, forming fat as a survival factor for hibernation. When spring comes, the vitamin D level rises, a normal metabolism sets in and the bear enjoy the summer in an active body.

The American Jeff Bowles writes in his remarkable book: *The miraculous effects of extremely high doses of Vitamin D3* of a similar hibernation syndrome in humans. If the vitamin D level drops, the mood also drops, depressive thoughts spread and the body demands a diet rich in fat and carbohydrates. Studies show that over-weight **persons and those** with inclination to depression have a very low D3 amount. In addition over-weight persons can utilize the vitamin D3 produced in the skin much less than slim persons. (66)

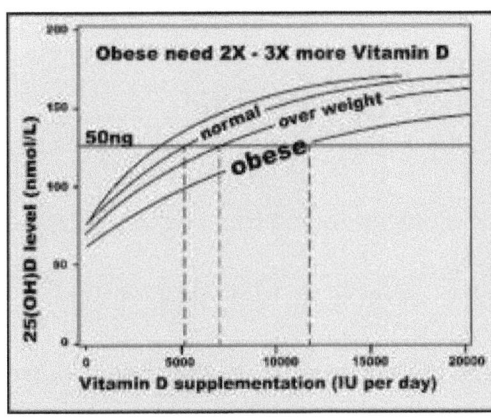

Source: vitaminwiki.com

Obesity is a chronic disease associated with excessive accumulation of fatty tissue in the body.

A 2014 study illustrates the relationship between body weight and vitamin D supplementation. The higher the body weight, the higher the vitamin D supplementation required. (67)

The low vitamin D values in blood tests are noticeable with obese persons. Overweight children in particular have inadequately low vitamin D levels.

The *Clinical Practice Guidelines* of the Endocrine Society recommend that doctors give overweight people two to three times more vitamin D than normal-weight people. "This is due to reduced bioavailability of Vitamin D in obesity." (68)

Obesity is often associated with little self-worth, self-love and tendency to depression. Vitamin D or UVB radiation has a brightening effect on the psyche. A weight-reducing measure is more promising once the person has gained a sufficient vitamin D supply.

Diabetes and vitamin D

Diabetes mellitus, also known as 'diabetes', is a chronic metabolic disease that manifests itself in an elevated blood sugar level.
There is a wealth of evidence that vitamin D stabilizes blood sugar metabolism in people with diabetes. In muscle, liver, pancreatic beta cells and insulin-producing cells, researchers have been able to demonstrate the effect. Vitamin D regulates excessive insulin secretion in cases of insulin resistance. (69)

Vitamin D in the metabolic system
- activates 1α-hydroxylase enzyme in pancreas, (70)
- increases insulin sensitivity by acting on muscle cell receptors, (71)
- strengthens cell-to-cell communication and thus regulates blood sugar in type 1 diabetes, (72)
- protects against irreversible defects in islet cells, insulin resistance and related defects. (70)
- Vitamin D deficiency influences glucose metabolism and is more important for diabetics than pure weight loss.

In 2011 *Nature Reviews Immunology* published a summary of the modulation of the immune system by UV radiation. The results clearly showed the relationship between vitamin D deficiency in insulin resistance and arterial hardening. "The two risk factors vitamin D deficiency and diabetes double the relative risk of developing cardiovascular disease. Even the mortality rate is higher in people with diabetes and vitamin D deficiency." (73)

Cholesterol and vitamin D

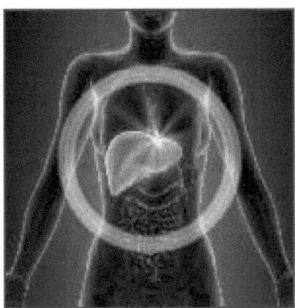

Cholesterol is a vital substance. It provides a flexible cell membrane and facilitates metabolic processes in the brain. It plays a decisive role in the formation of vitamin D and certain hormones. Since cholesterol is a precursor of vitamin D, inhibition of the synthesis of cholesterol (e.g. by cholesterol inhibitors) also prevents the synthesis of vitamin D. Cholesterol is essential for vitamin D synthesis by sunlight.

(74)

In 2013, researchers led by Pamela Lindsey discovered a link between calcium and vitamin D intake. They report improved cholesterol levels in obese menopausal women by taking these two supplements. (75)

In a study by Cutillas-Marco E. et al. further scientists found a connection between vitamin D and cholesterol. They concluded that "a higher level of vitamin D reduces the level of cholesterol in the blood and reduces the risk of cardiovascular disease". At high cholesterol levels, serum traces of vitamin D were lower. (76)

Extensive further studies in the field of metabolism and vitamin D come to analogous results:
Metabolic syndrome, Crohn's disease, arthritis, periodontitis, thyroid disorders, gout, rheumatism and more. (34)

Cardiovascular system and the photon carrier vitamin D

When several systems are in disorder, a body reacts differently for each individual person. These disorders could affect the heart and circulation.

All disturbances of the cardiovascular system come from the specific aspects of the systems and are therefore caused individually. At the cellular level, a disturbed information and communication field occurs due to a lack of light or, more clearly, due to a lack of photons.

Numerous indications of a special vitamin D protective function are:
- Vitamin D is associated with cardiovascular disease factors.
- Vitamin D is involved in the regulation of blood pressure (e.g. in hypertension).
- Vitamin D is effective against chronic inflammations.
- Vitamin D protects blood vessels and the heart muscle directly.

An extensive study, published in the *ÄrzteZeitung* in 2012, comes to the conclusion that "a low vitamin D level increases the risk of getting coronary heart disease or a heart attack". (77) Not surprising is the bone loss in congestive heart failure. (78)

High blood pressure and Vitamin D

A major risk factor for cardiovascular diseases is high blood pressure, hypertension.

In a double-blind study, Danish researchers established the link between cardiovascular mortality in hypertensive patients, vitamin D and high blood pressure. The results of the observational study suggest that a low vitamin D level is one of the causes of certain heart diseases. The medical journal reported on this NHANES study on 14 May 2012 and commented: "Hypertensives significantly lowered their central blood pressure if they substituted vitamin D in the winter months. (79)

Mortality risk reduced with Vitamin D

Vitamin D deficiency is not only causally involved in cardiovascular diseases, but also increases the risk of a premature death from this disease. A meta-analysis with 6,853 patients with cardiovascular disease showed "that the mortality risk decreases by 14% by increasing the 25 (OH) D levels". (80) Further studies with similar results are available. (81)

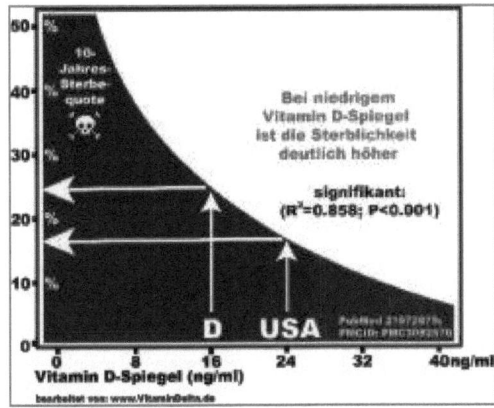

The scientists around Prof. Dr. Karin Amrein, Clinical Department of Endocrinology and Metabolism at the Medical University of Graz, made an amazing discovery. "Seriously ill patients, who exhibited a strongly lowered vitamin D value at the beginning of the study were treated with the high-dose vitamin D3. This resulted in a clearly low mortality rate in comparison to the control group. Karin Amrein: "Our study is the first major study of vitamin D in intensive care units worldwide. A vitamin D level determination should be established for critically ill patients, since vitamin D intake appears to reduce mortality in cases of severe vitamin D deficiency. (82)

Atherosclerosis and vitamin D

Atherosclerosis belongs to the group of arteriosclerosis, also is known as arteriosclerosis or the hardening of the arteries. It is a systemic disease of the arteries that leads to deposits of blood lipids, thrombus, connective tissue and, to a lesser extent, calcium in the vascular walls. The *Journal of clinical laboratory* analytics published a study in 2015 (83) with the result: "Vitamin D can reduce inflammation and resolve arterial stiffness in arteriosclerosis". (84)

Vitamin D deficiency can also inhibit the synthesis of various vascular-protective substances such as interleukin 10, matrix Gla protein, osteopontin and type IV collagen.

Cancer and vitamin D

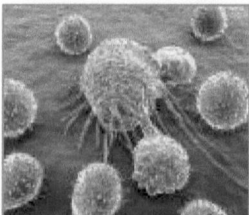

All 700 billion cells in our body perform their own tasks according to their genetic imprint. Almost all cell types in the human body change constantly, they die and new cells are built.

A controlled death (apoptosis) regulates the cell division and renewal process. Disturbances in the controlled dying of the cells are associated with the development of numerous diseases such as cancer, diabetes or Alzheimer's disease.

Cancer develops in several steps. (85) Cancer cells are extremely versatile. They develop in the individual aspects of the systems. They can adapt to new conditions in a very short time by constantly changing the genetic material. Cancer develops when the body's own cells divide independently, progressively and excessively. "This is a matter of biophotonic light intensity. Prof. Dr. Popp says that cancer is caused by a lack of light. (5)

All types of cancer are obviously caused by insufficient vitamin D intake or production. This is seen as a co-factor in the development of a disease. (86)

Insufficient vitamin D levels are associated with ovarian cancer, (87) polycystic ovary syndrome (88), rheumatoid arthritis (89), lupus erythematosus and other conditions. (90)

Breast cancer and vitamin D

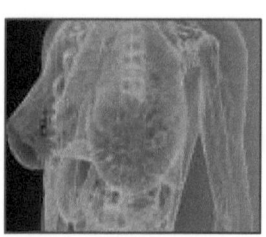

Breast cancer is the most commonly diagnosed cancer among women in Western industrialized countries, but not the most dangerous.

Harvard University in Boston conducted a large-scale study of 50,000 nurses and 22,000 doctors. This study, known as the 'Nurse Study', found a 30 percent lower risk of breast cancer with sufficient vitamin D levels. Furthermore all three studies showed a slight protection from pancreatic cancer. (48)

PLOS ONE published a cohort study from the year 2016. (91) Scientists found that women over 55 with blood concentrations of vitamin D higher than 40 ng/ml had a 67% lower risk of cancer compared to women with a level below 20 ng/ml.

The organization *Breastcancer* in Ardmore PA, USA recommends women to take a vitamin D supplementation. "A vitamin D supplement might even be able to stop breast cancer cells from developing." (92)

Colitis and vitamin D

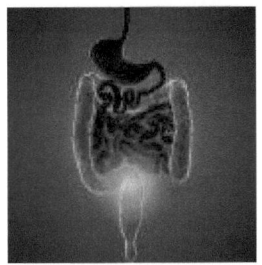

Ulcerative colitis is a chronic inflammatory disease of the large intestine, usually in episodes, which often originates in the rectum and can spread to the entire large intestine.

Researchers from Beth Israel Deaconess Medical Center (BIDMC) - one of Harvard University's teaching hospitals - found that lower vitamin D levels in the blood increase the risk of relapse in patients with ulcerative colitis. Low levels of vitamin D are regularly measured in patients with active ulcerative colitis. It was so far unclear whether these low values could also enforce the danger of the active phase. (93) This will be the subject of another study.

The *American Journal of Clinical Nutrition* published a study in July 2016 that also showed the relationship between low vitamin D levels and increased colitis activity. In addition, a connection was found between the level of vitamin D and the severity of the disease and relapse in patients with inflammatory bowel disease. (94)

Higher life expectancy and vitamin D

The results of a study published in July 2014 showed that "cancer patients with higher vitamin D levels between 75 and 30 ng/ml had better chances of survival and lived longer than patients with vitamin D status lower than 30 ng/ml". (95)

Vitamin D as photon carrier:
- controls cell division, cell growth, cell death and cell cycle,
- supports proper cell-to-cell communication, (96)
- enables the cells to recognize and dispose of malignant cells, (97)
- acts as an immune system modulator, (96)
- prevents excessive production of inflammatory cytokines and increases macrophage activity,
- stimulates the production of strong anti-microbial peptides in other white blood cells and epithelial cells, (98)
- protects organs from infection. (29)

"Our goal was to determine the levels of vitamin D that can prevent the development of invasive, previously known cancers," said Cedric Garland in 2016, researcher and adjunct professor at the UC San Diego School of Medicine, Department of Family Medicine and Public Health. He concluded that optimal vitamin D levels for cancer prevention "range between 40 and 60 ng/ml. Most cancers occur in people with vitamin D blood levels between 10 and 40 ng/ml." (99)

Life activities and the photon carrier vitamin D

Pregnancy and vitamin D

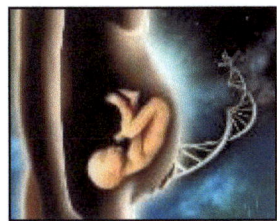 Every pregnancy is an enigma for mother and child. A constant process of growth and division is going on. After fertilization a single cell becomes a perfect human being with billions of cells. Each of these cells performs a specific function in the body. It retains the characteristics of the original cell from which it originated from. When these unimaginably complex processes take place in a precise and photon-rich order matrix, the mother and child start a healthy, happy life. The greater the order of the fields, the greater the chance for the body and life to be in optimal balance.

Vitamin D, often referred to as the love hormone, plays a key role in pregnancy. Vitamin receptors are found in amniotic fluid, uterus and embryonic stem cells. Recent studies show the connections between maternal vitamin D status and the structure of the fetal skeleton or the formation of the immune and nervous systems. Mental and physical health in later life also depend on a sufficient supply of vitamin D during pregnancy.

The magazine *Woman's Health* published a study in 2012, which confirmed the contraction strength of the uterine muscle by vitamin D receptors there. The study spoke of "immuno-modulatory effects of vitamin D in pregnancy". This is considered a potential protection for the mother against infections. (100)

A good supply of vitamin D in the womb lays important foundations not only until the birth but also for the health of the child throughout life. (101)
"Vitamin D plays a central role in the epigenetic imprinting of the child", confirms the physician and researcher Lapilonne from Paris Descartes University, Paris (France).

Dr. Lisa Bodnar, a vitamin D researcher at the University of Pittsburgh, believes that "a vitamin D deficiency during pregnancy endangers the life and health of the mother. It is one of the causes of future threats to the child, especially to the brain and immune system." (102)

Dr. Dijkstra and his colleagues studied 70 pregnant women in the Netherlands, "none of them had a vitamin D level above 40 ng/ml. 50% had values below 10 ng/ml. Again, prenatal vitamins had little effect on 25 (OH) D levels. Prenatal vitamins contain only 400 I.E. vitamin D. This by far did not satisfy the requirements of a pregnant woman." (103)

Further studies associated with vitamin D confirm the important role of the vitamin before, during and after pregnancy. Pregnancy planning, gestational diabetes, pre-eclampsia or pregnancy poisoning, bacterial vaginitis, caesarean section, birth weight, MS and pregnancy depression were the subject of various studies. (34)

Vitamin D as carrier of photons is important for mother and unborn
- healthy development of the placenta,
- extensive unfolding of the brain,
- precise defense mechanisms of the immune system,
- fine formation of organs, skeletons and systems
- special intelligence of the child,
- predisposition to certain autoimmune diseases,
- conscious gene activity (epigenetics), (104)

Eye Health and vitamin D

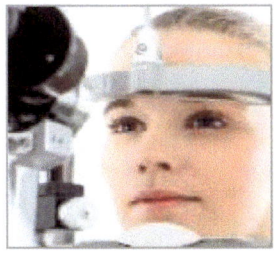

Vitamin D protects the eyes from premature aging, including inflammation. (105)

Scientists confirm: „already a six-week dose of vitamin D improved vision in middle-aged people." (106)

Professor Glen Jeffery, of University College London, said in 2012: "There is increasing evidence that many of us are already suffering from age-related inflammation and retinal damage, including macular degeneration, due to insufficient vitamin D supply. (107)

Athletes and Vitamin D

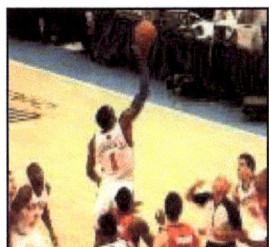

Vitamin D plays an important role for athletes. The stability and flexibility of the bone mass, as well as the immunity, the endurance and the physical capacity are decisive.

Alexander, a graduate sports scientist, is convinced that "Vitamin D can play a decisive role when it comes to promoting muscle/bone growth and increasing testosterone levels as well as the entire immune system in recreational, amateur and competitive sports". (108) "No matter what kind of sport we do the human skeleton and muscles have to be exposed to the permanent interactions between tension, pressure, rotation and shearing movements. Vitamin D ensures these coordinated interactions."

"Vitamin D improves the resilience and performance of the heart-lung system, promotes muscle growth, increases maximum oxygen uptake, reduces the degree of inflammation of the muscular tissue, strengthens the heart-lung system and increases testosterone production. (109)

Pineal gland and vitamin D

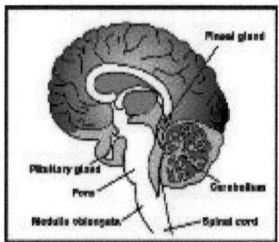

Sunlight affects the pineal gland. The glandula pinealis is the pineal gland or epiphysis. It is connected to the third eye, the gate to God or the 6th seal.

It is a small pine cone-shaped organ in the brain that secretes hormones such as melatonin, serotonin and DMT (dimethyltryptamine). Melatonin is responsible for a relaxed sleep cycle and for meditative and emotional states of well-being. It has an extraordinarily strong antioxidant potential which repairs cell damage.

Serotonin is known as the happiness hormone because it has a relaxing and highly mood-lifting effect.

Modern lifestyle leads to a shrinking of the pineal gland. The organ shrinks from its original size of approx. 3 centimeters to a few millimeters. If the function of the pineal gland decreases, the physical and psychological aging process begins. (110)

In addition, increasingly higher loads of various toxins cause the gland to calcify. Fluorides and mercury are among them.

Based on research results, more pineal calcifications occur in Alzheimer patients than in people with other forms of dementia. Both have a vitamin D and a melatonin deficiency situation in common. (111) Vitamin D as a fat-soluble hormone regulates the calcium metabolism and stimulates the pineal gland. Dr. David William describes Vitamin D as 'decalcifyer of the pineal gland'. (341)

Older people live better with vitamin D

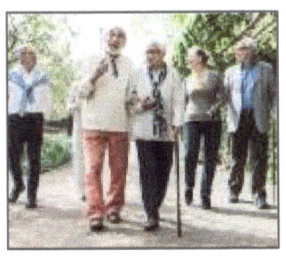

Studies show that all seniors over 65 benefit from vitamin D supplementation. Health aspects, increased vitality and active physical and mental participation in life improve.

A new study under the direction of Dr. Barbara Boucher now propagates a vitamin D supplementation for women after menopause, i.e. from about 50, of double the dose. "The goal for these women must be a blood serum value of 40 ng/ml," says the scientist. (112)

Aging slows down metabolic processes and also leads to a reduced ability to produce vitamin D in the skin. A 70-year-old person who is exposed to the same sun as a 20-year-old produces only about 25% of the vitamin D that a 20-year-old can produce. (113)

In particular, mobility is often reduced with increasing age. The risk of progressive osteoporosis is increased. This can lead to falls and fractures with severe consequences. Dr. Barbara Boucher confirmed this in her 2012 study. (114)

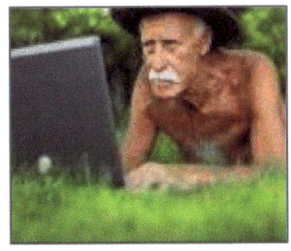

Heike Bischoff-Ferrari, Professor of Geriatrics at the University of Zurich, was able to prove in 2010 that seniors who took a high dose of vitamin D daily after a hip fracture were less frequently admitted to hospital in the following year than the peer group. The journalist Marita Fuchs reported about this for the University of Zurich. (115)

Research conducted by the Buck Institute for research on aging in October 2016 showed that vitamin D worked in precisely those genes associated with longevity. Vitamin D as sun-hormone also influences all processes associated with the development of age-related diseases. Professor Gordon Lithgow of the Buck Institute established that "Vitamin D in the longevity genes prolongs the average lifespan of proteins by 33 percent and at the same time slows down age-related deficiency development". (116)

Younger, healthier and fitter with vitamin D

Chromosomes are the carriers of genetic material. This genetic material determines how an organism develops. "Telomeres are the ends of our genetic material threads, the chromosomes. They serve as protective caps. With each cell division, they become a little shorter," explains Blackurn, one of the discoverers of telomeres and Nobel Prize winner of 2009 in an interview with the Network for Ageing Research (NAR). If the critical length of the cell is undercut as a result of this shortening, the cell undergoes an ageing process and cell death. The cell becomes "inoperative". (117) If the cell remains healthy and capable of action for a long time, it will divide less frequently. This is the prominence of life. Biophotons in vitamin D produce their own enzyme, telomerase, to stimulate telomere growth.

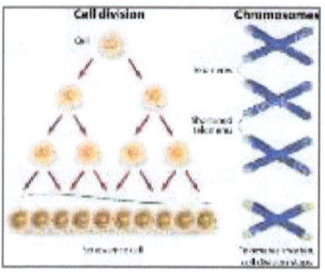

Mira Mamtani reports of a large-scale study from 2016. (118) Scientists, inspired by the newest realizations searched to what extent vitamin D values in the serum actually affect the telomere growth. This study, known as the National Health and Nutrition Examination Survey, showed "a possible positive association between vitamin D status and telomere length". (119) Vitamin D seems to ensure cell activity in perfect order.

DNA, life's building plan and vitamin D

DNA is the conductor, architect and mediator of genetic messages to all cells of our body. It contains the genetic code for every aspect, and every potential, of our entire life. (120)

Let us remember that billions of photon-stimulated-communications take place per second in the body and precisely secure these complex networks.

Vitamin D as a photon carrier:
- offers protection against oxidative DNA damage, (121)
- precisely regulates the growth and cell division rate of the cells, (122)
- prevents damage to DNA,
- offers protection against carcinogenesis, (121)
- allows the experience of greater potentials,
- opens channels for communication to other levels of perception.

The innate ability of gene repair opens up an inexhaustible potential for human beings to perceive themselves as co-creators.

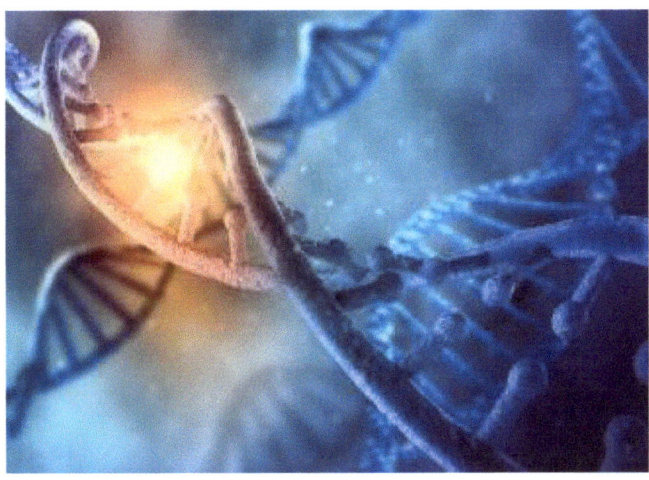

More Vitamin D is needed for all those persons:
- with dark skin,
- in sunshine poor regions,
- with liver, kidney and bowel health problems,
- with obesity and anorexia,
- with high toxin loads such as DDT, PCB,
- with increased alcohol and nicotine consumption,
- with osteoporosis and other bone metabolic disorders,
- with a lack of cofactors such as magnesium, vitamin K2 and omega-3,
- after surgery, chemotherapy or trauma,
- with mental and psychological stress,
- those, who take drugs or Vitamin D reducing drugs - like statins
- during and after pregnancy,
- in advanced age,
- with increased physical demands, such as athletes and physical heavy labor,
- in exam situations and in major decision-makings.

Blood – the bridge into life

Fourth week of pregnancy. A diligent growth and cell division takes place in the uterus. The small embryo already measures a few millimeters. Its tiny body is transparent and gelatinous. Even before the heart of the embryo beats, blood forms. Only then does the heart develop.

Blood is the data highway into all visible and invisible aspects. Blood shows like no other organ that every cell is penetrated by light, i.e. by consciousness.

Sweat blood and tears
Music is in her blood.
Bad blood
between the two families
Blood is thicker than water
Make (someone's) blood boil
Blue blood in noble or aristocratic family

These idioms show emotional, individually felt experiences. Blood is the fastest perceivable, photon-excited reaction field in the organism.

In modern medicine, comprehensive, technical blood analyses are the means of diagnosis and treatment. The laboratory proceeds meticulously. Sir Isaac Newton, father of classical physics, would be delighted. Just like the laboratory computers, he would measure, count, weigh, observe and precisely define the ratio of small to large blood cells in pikograms. David Bohm the quantum physicists would look for the causative potentials already from the quantum level - holistically. For him it is self-evident that consciousness (information) and energy create reality. Thoughts influence blood values.

Practice proves it

Some blood values drastically worsen from an emotional experience. Once the crisis or conflict has been overcome, this can also be seen in the physical blood improvement.

Blood values are more than a column of numbers. They provide us with information about the degree of our well-being and point to possible disturbances in the metabolism or other systems. Blood values provide information about emotions, talents, strengths, inclinations and thus help to set valuable cognitive processes in motion. (123)

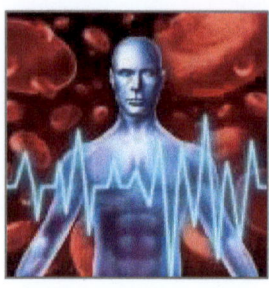 Blood not only stores all the vital information that characterizes a person and makes him a unique personality, it also moves this information in a constant, rhythmic cycle. Blood reaches along its 150,000 kilometers bloodlines every corner of the body, no matter how remote. It serves as a sophisticated garbage disposal system, it defends, and supplies the entire system. Communication, however, which organizes and controls this exchange is located on a completely different level - that of light. It is an interaction of light and matter. The transmitter of communication and drive is ensured by photons. The same is displayed by all body fluids, especially water.

Blood is the bridge connecting all organs with each other and bears eloquent witness to the miracle of life.

Blood sings and moves in the rhythm of life.

PART 3
The Creative Bridge

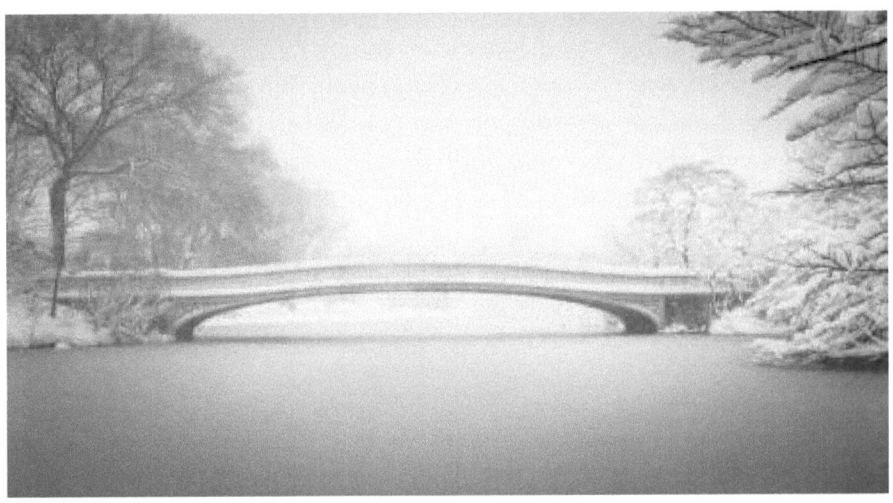

If we understand this 'bridge', we have the key to our health in our hands.

Bridges are omnipresent in nature, in our bodies and in creation. Bridges connect, from one side to the other, from one state to another. The essential bridges are invisible to the human eye.

We always experience ourselves as a whole being. Only when dysfunctions occur do we perceive this disturbed part of our organism as a part that stands alone, such as a sick liver or a weak thyroid gland.

It is the quantum physics that provides us with new insights.
Sir Isaac Newton, the father of science (1642 – 1726) did what we continue to do most of these days. He observed the everyday world and searched for explanations and laws. Everyday world is what we see, weigh, measure, and calculate - one separate from the other.
As a physicist, he endeavored to describe natural processes as generally as possible. This means that the laws should be formulated in such a way

that they are as independent as possible from the point of view of the observer. The laws of nature should be independent to the observer, i.e. to the human being. Physics is the science of material objects.

At the beginning of the 20th century David Bohm, a quantum physicist showed that in addition to the world of things familiar and visible to us, there is another realm of reality in which everything is not arbitrary but exactly mathematical, interwoven and connected with everything else. It forms an indivisible wholeness and thus represents a more fundamental aspect. Only about 1 to 7% of reality lies in the visible range.

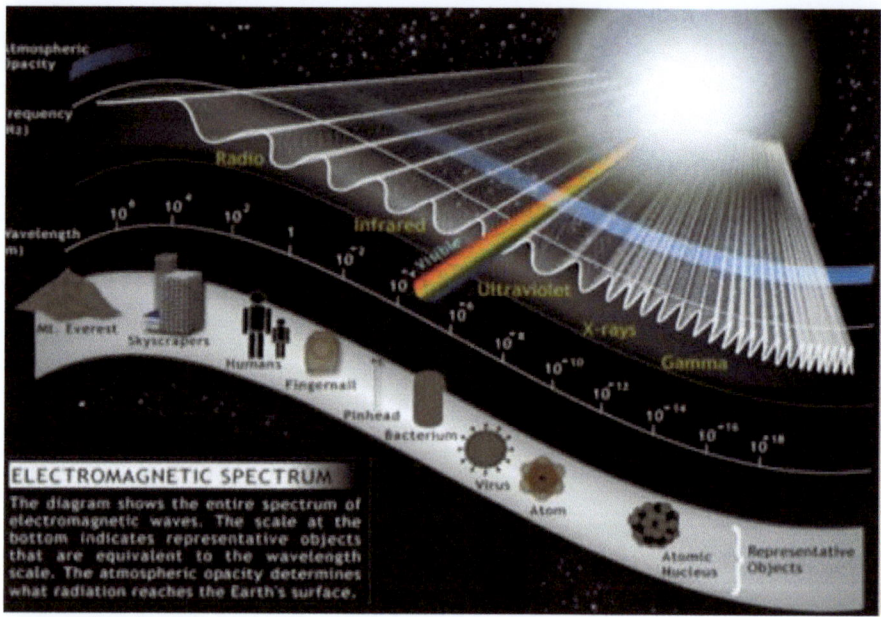

Source. (124)

In quantum physics, space and time take on completely new dimensions. Dimensions, some of which exist only on paper, because never before has a human being seen them, yet dreamed them and considered them possible. Quantum physics deals with the behavior of the smallest particles, the quanta and their interactions. These quanta are invisible to the human eye.

There must be something that connects the visible with the invisible.

All that appears separately is one
Let's take a closer look:

DNA - the genotype
Data unmodifiable
All structure and functional data of a human being
Coherent, in order
> #### DNA - The individual phenotype
> Data modifiable, individual
> Genetically influenced from the maternal and paternal line
> Incoherent, out of order

Immune system - autonomous, innate
Data unalterable - fixed in the genome
Ordered defense system
Coherent, in order
> #### Immune system - individually acquired
> Data alterable, acquired immune system
> Immune defense develops only in the course of life,
> Incoherent, out of order

Nervous system - autonomous, innate
Unalterable vital bodily functions such as heartbeat,
Respiration, blood pressure, digestion and metabolism. Coherent
> #### Nervous system - somatic, individual
> Data can be changed, reacts to individual experiences
> Fight Flight System,
> Incoherent, out of order

Metabolism - autonomous
Data cannot be changed, all information for a
Optimal, healthy, active, future-oriented life
Coherent, in order
> #### Metabolism - somatic or psychological
> Data can be changed, individual
> Reacts to life experiences, food and environmental facts,
> Incoherent, out of order

We live with these two equal systems in one polarity. If we were to choose only the autonomous, optimal aspect, it would be boring. Every human being would be equal, without individuality, without a special uniqueness that makes us attractive and admirable. No challenge to explore life with our own talents and strengths. There would be no evolution.

Only the individual system gives us the freedom to diversify. We humans define ourselves mostly due to individual presetting, life circumstances, illnesses, conflicts, education exclusively with the individual part. Our inherent limitations and emotions such as lack, fear and insecurity also demand energy in the form of photons or light. Ultimately this leads to an aging process based on lack of light.

When both types, as medicine says, are inseparably connected with each other, then there should also be 'bridges'. These bridges would allow the transfer of data to restore the light balance, healing information, or other desired information.

Actually - these bridges exist - and they are scientifically proven.

They seem invisible to the naked eye. They are only detectable by their effect.

Take water as an example: Water looks like water to the naked eye. The hidden life of water lies in the invisible. Prof. Pollack discovered this secret and discovered a fourth state, the intermediate medium or exclusion zone.

The Bridge-Medium – the connecting medium

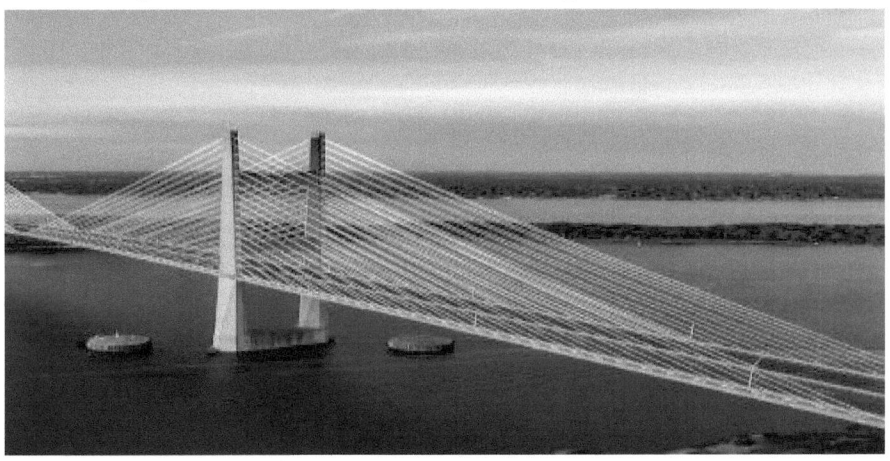

In his laboratory in Seattle (USA), Dr. Gerald Pollack, Professor of Bioengineering, and his team discovered such a 'bridge' or transition stage in water.

Basic chemistry teaches us that water appears in three states or phases: solid, liquid and gas. But when Pollack started to treat the water with light, he discovered another state. He called this fourth phase the exclusion zone (EZ). This zone acts as a bridge-medium.

When we freeze water it goes from regular water to EZ water then to ice. And when we melt it, it changes from ice to EZ water and back to regular water. So EZ water is an intermediate or bridge building state. (125)

"In our laboratory at the University of Washington, we've done many experiments over the last decade. These experiments have clearly shown the existence of this additional phase of water." (125)

According to Pollack, there's compelling evidence that EZ water is indeed lifesaving. (126)

"The key ingredient to create exclusion zone water is light; i.e., electro-magnetic energy, whether in the form of visible light, ultraviolet (UV) wavelengths and infrared wavelengths, which we are surrounded by all the time." (126)

The gel-like exclusion zones are charged, which means they carry potential energy. "This charge can be used," Pollack says, "to stimulate all cellular processes from chemical reactions to blood flow. (123)
Is energy lacking, the exclusion zone or the bridge medium begins to dissolve. Without sufficient radiant energy, the growth and separation process reverses and the battery discharges.

This honeycomb shaped, liquid-crystal-bridge plays an important role in all aspects of human life, since humans are "water beings".

No life would be possible without this active in-between-medium in the body. The more potent and transmitting this medium is, the healthier and vital life is.

Pollack describes this zone as the motor of life, generated by light. (126)
The ideal light sources are coming from the UVB radiance of the sun and of course the Blu Room.
Chlorophyll, vitamin D, c60 act as the purest photonic batteries.

The UVB frequency in the atmosphere of the Blu Room generates perfect structured water.
Masaru Emoto, physician of naturopathy, developed a method to make frequencies in water memorably visible. He is convinced: "Everything in the universe vibrates. The highest vibrational frequency is the frequency of unconditional love. Fear, on the other hand, vibrates at the lowest frequency." (127)

Water crystals with structured water from the Blu Room BluRelax, Klagenfurt, Austria give a beautiful testimony.

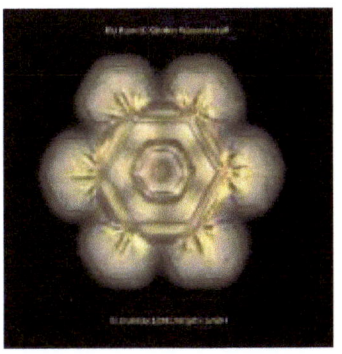 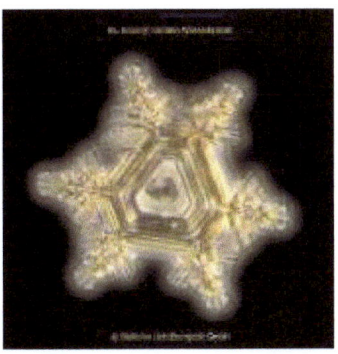

Here are some crystal pictures from Blu Room Salamander, Kaegiswil, Switzerland.

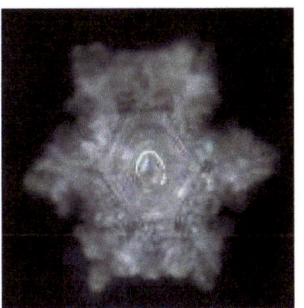 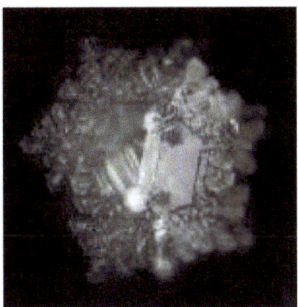 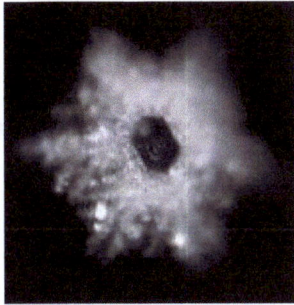

The left one is Blu Room water standing on Flower of Life symbol.
The middle one is Blu Room water standing on salamander logo.
The picture to the right is pure tap water in Kägiswil.

UVB-Light – photonic wealth

In 1801 Johann Wilhelm Ritter discovered an invisible light beyond the violet end of the light spectrum, the ultraviolet light. (128)

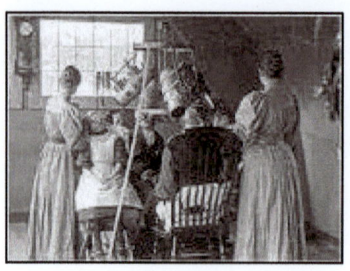

Thereafter numerous scientists experimented with these new rays.

In 1896, Niels Ryberg Finsen, the father of ultraviolet therapy, developed the first bacteria-destroying lamp. With this Finsen lamp he treated over 800 people suffering under lupus vulgaris. The success rates were 98%. Lupus vulgaris is the most common form of skin tuberculosis. In 1901 he received the Nobel Prize for his outstanding services. (129)

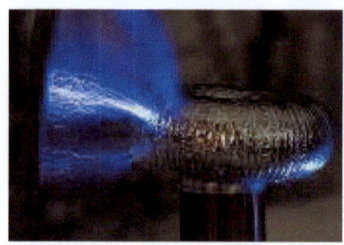

In 1891 the inventor Nikola Tesla designed a resonance transformer, also known as a Tesla coil. This coil generates UV waves of considerable power. With this blue light radiating device he also introduced a certain form of frequency therapy. (130)

Source: teslasociety.com

In his book *Cross Currents: The Perils of Electropollution, the Promise of Electromedicine* (1994), published in 1990, Dr. Robert Becker describes numerous healing experiences with the Tesla coil. The healing of cancer is documented under the title: "Lightning struck the chin: cancer disappeared in two weeks", "breast tumor diminished".

This frequency therapy also accelerated the elimination of waste products out of the blood. All this contributed to healing. (131)

The research results of these two doctors Virgil Hancock and Emmet K. Knott published in the book *Education of Cancer Healing* in 1942 show the following experiences with photoluminescence therapy (UV light therapy):

- Inactivation of toxins
- Destruction and inhibition of bacterial growth
- Better blood and oxygen transport to the organs
- Stimulation of cellular and humoral immunity
- Activation of steroid hormones
- Vasodilatation, (dilatation of blood vessels)
- Activation of white blood cells
- Reduced platelet aggregation (thrombosis protection)
- Stimulation of fibrinolysis (breakdown of blood clots)
- Reduced viscosity of blood
- Stimulation of corticosteroid production. (Corticosteroids, or corticosteroids, are steroid hormones synthesized from cholesterol in the adrenal cortex.)
- Improved microcirculation (132)

The two doctors treated 6,800 patients with UV therapy. Not a single patient complained of side effects. (133)

William Campbell Douglass, MD, author of the book *Into the Light – The Medicine of the Future* Today travelled the world, marching to the coldest regions of Siberia, South Africa, the USA and Europe to garner the experience of doctors who had very good results with UV light even in the most difficult situations.

Somewhat frustrated, Douglass notes at the end of his book: "It is unimaginable that the best solution to stop worldwide 'killer diseases' is ignored, despised and discarded." (134)

Many of his reports are presented in detail in the master book *Blu Room – experience the future*. (34) Here is a small excerpt:

Bacterial endocarditis: Patients received two to three UV light treatments per day. 60% of the patients were discharged after a short time. It was noticeable that the hospital stay was significantly shortened. In addition, the two doctors were able to determine a recovery time after coma twice as fast when the persons were irradiated with UV light. (134)

UV light and blood poisoning: Ukrainian doctors confirmed a "rapid disappearance of poisoning symptoms and fever after blood irradiation with UV light." (134)

UV Light and food poisoning: Miley reported in the *Archives of Physical Therapy*, Volume 25, June 1944, the case of a patient with life-threatening food poisoning caused by botulinum toxin. They treated his blood with UV light. Within 48 hours he could swallow and had regained his eyesight.

UV light and pneumonia: Patients with "advanced pneumonia, acute gangrenous appendicitis, multiple pelvic abscesses and peritonitis were out of the critical, life-threatening situation and on their way to recovery within 24 to 72 hours". (134)

UV light and coronary arteries: A group of St. Petersburg physicians tested the effect of photoluminescence in 145 patients. "137 of the 145 patients treated with UV light therapy showed a significant improvement within a short time. A rapid pain reduction was noticeable; the use of analgesics (pain killers) could be discontinued. Angina pectoris attacks were far less frequent than in patients treated with conventional drugs." (134)

UV light and military: During the Second World War, American and Russian troops used UV light irradiation for disinfection, food preservation and medical applications. (134)

UV light and convalescence: Based on his extensive experience, Campbell noted that the general condition of the patients improved almost immediately after the first treatment. Appetite increased and hope returned. "Remarkable," says Campbell, "is the rapid recovery of a weakened body and increased self-regulation in UV light therapy (photoluminescence)." (134)

UV light and gout: After UV irradiation, the body can regulate uric acid more quickly and excrete it. Doctors observed this effect not only in patients with gout, but also in people with arthritis or bursitis. (134)

In recent decades, the industry has been inspired by these successes to innovative machines and systems:

- In September 2006, the world's largest UV drinking water disinfection plant with a capacity of 2.5 million m3 per day was opened in St. Petersburg, Russia. (135)
- Air conditioning systems with UV light filters kill organic substances such as bacteria, mold and viruses. UV light penetrates through the thin cell membrane membranes of these organisms and inactivates their DNA. (136)
- In washing machines and dishwashers, UV light ensures sterile laundry or dishes.
- A UV light comb slows down the rapid, abnormal cell division in psoriasis. The disease hotspots heal gradually under constant treatment.
- Blue light emitting brooms disinfect hospital corridors

- Entire operating rooms are clinically clean. A radiation system floods hospital rooms with intensive millisecond pulses of ultraviolet light. (468) UVC radiation alters the DNA of microorganisms in such a way that reproduction is no longer possible.
- 2017 A UV light pyjama treats babies suffering from jaundice after birth "The photonic textiles are washable and well tolerated by the skin", says the EMPA research team around Maike Quandt and Luciano. (137)

Accelerated relaxation
2017 Researchers at the University of Granada confirm accelerated relaxation after high stress exposure under UV light compared to conventional white light. (138)

Faster thanks to blue light
2017 Researchers of the University of Basel have confirmed in a study with 74 male athletes: Athletes who expose themselves to blue light before a competition in the evening can significantly improve in the final sprint. (139)

UVB - promising in chronic kidney disease
In January 2017, the *International Journal of Nephrology and Renovascular Disease* published a study on treatment options for chronic kidney disease. The scientists concluded that "UVB light therapy and GLA are promising for the treatment of chronic kidney disease". (140)

UVB light treatments heal wounds faster
UVB light treatment before surgery requires less anesthesia, accelerates wound healing, prevents infection and reduces postoperative pain. (141) A discharge from the hospital is quicker with minimal complications. (134)

Blue light helps in later stages of wound healing
2018 Several institutes are currently developing high-tech patch pads that can heal wounds faster with light and also monitor healing. As part of the EU Medilight project, the CSEM research institute in Neuchâtel and six partners have developed a portable device for the treatment of chronic wounds. (142)

2015 Patent application filed for the world's first Blu Room® with innovative UVB technology.

2016 Blu Room–treatments begin
In January 2016, doctors at the Absolute Health Clinic in Olympia, WA, led by Dr. Matthew Martinez, began using Blu Room technology.

2018 Patent granted for the Blu Room®
The inventor Judith Darlene Knight was granted a patent on the 20th of March 2018 under the number US 9,919,162 for a device for light therapy.

> The patent document states:
> „Methods and apparatuses for providing therapy, including light therapy, to a user positioned within an enclosure are described herein. A method includes generating and selecting therapy settings based on user information and positioning the user within an enclosure having a plurality of light sources. " (183)

"I refuse to let anything blind me to possibilities"
JZ Knight

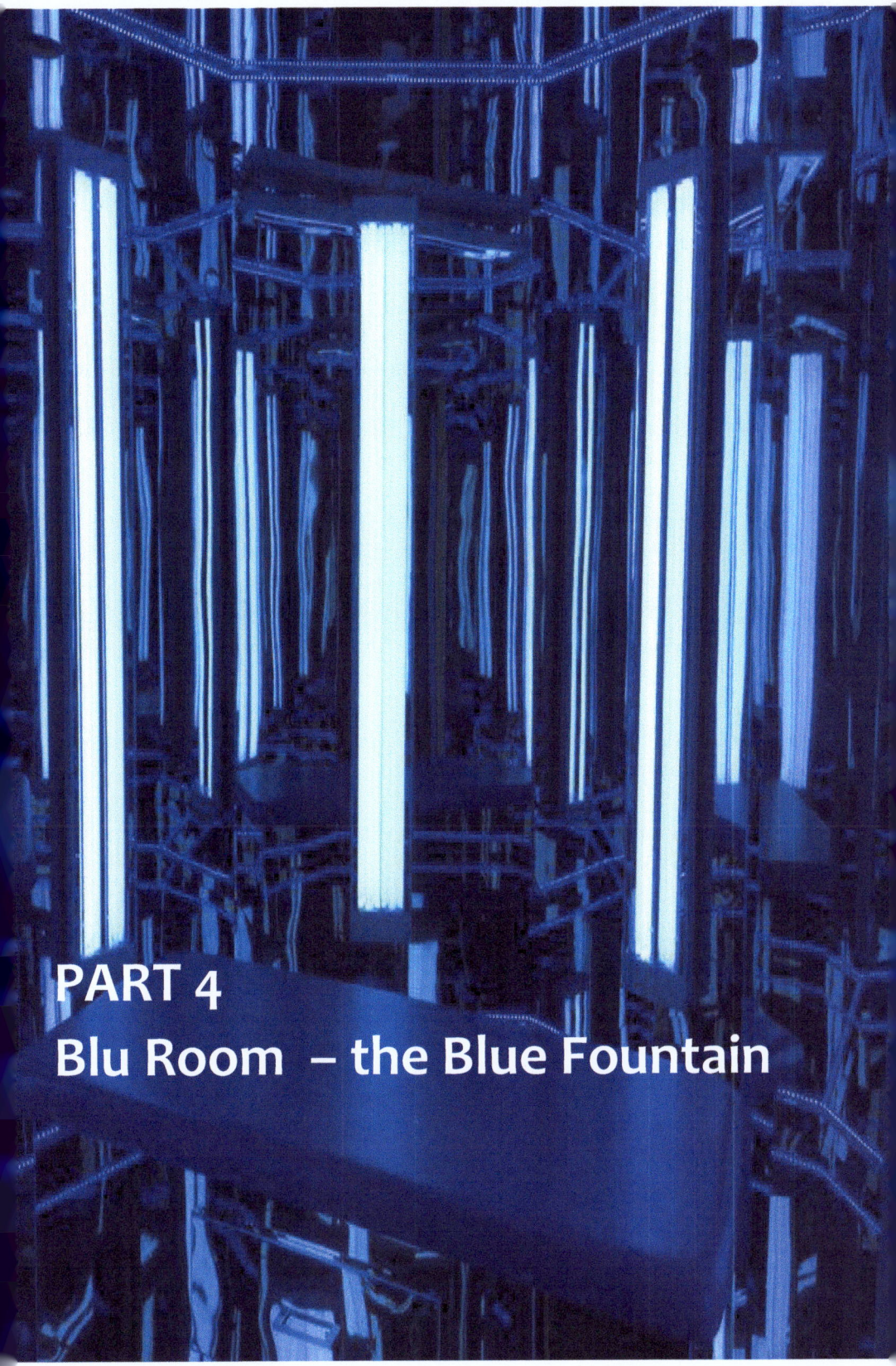

PART 4
Blu Room – the Blue Fountain

Warm, gentle, peaceful, magical, elegant, touching - these are the first impressions when the door to the Blu Room opens and the blue, warm light releases the brilliant architecture with its mirrored surfaces. Beauty and elegance in its purest form.

> The door to the Blu Room closes. The outside world is faded out. My body on the couch feels like on a white, warm sandy beach. The sound of the music weaves through the room, the waves reflect, meet again in the center, flow out once more, reflect anew and thus keep up the pulse of life in the highest order. A last look upwards into the mirrored ceiling. The blue LEDs stimulate an image of infinity. Then safety glasses over the eyes and simply sink into the surface. Now the UVB tubes begin to radiate. Soothing warmness permeates my cells. The invisible begins to work. I feel safe in this atmosphere, protected, carried, loved and strengthened. My body seems to get an 'update', new stimulus regarding the situation it is in and the corrections that are needed.

Perfect architecture, subtle sound, soft light and regulating frequencies create a protective atmosphere of deep calm, order and freedom.

Blu Room is far more than just the latest UVB-technology.
Seattle Newspaper journalist Michael Schindler described the Blu Room as a technology that "shields you from the outside world and wraps you in an atmosphere of soft ultraviolet light. Since your brain isn't busy responding to the stimulus of the everyday environment, your mind is free to relax or hold a relaxed state of focus without distractions." (143)

Octogon – the final balance

This impressive geometric shape of the octogon in the Blu Room seems like a timeless merging of human history.

Since ancient times, the octogon has had a symbolic significance that goes back to the archetype of the eight-pointed star. It expresses:

- Perfection
- Regeneration
- Wholeness
- Infinity
- Rebirth
- Transition (144)

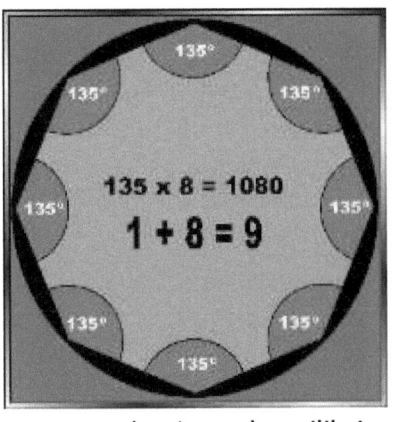

Old philosophies regard the octogon "as the final balance between matter and invisible forces, the complete balance between material and spiritual, heart and mind, inhalation as well as exhalation of the Creator and creation. (145)

The Greek philosopher Pythagoras was convinced that the "eightness of the octogon is like the embrace of heavenly harmony". He tied it to security, constancy and universal equilibrium.

From the perspective of the Sumerians, the octogon is the realization of the number nine. The digits of one angle with 135° sum up to 9. The digit sum of all eight angles together results in 9.

Perfection – no beginning and no end.

Nine is according to ancient Vedas the number of perfection and divine symmetry

In 2008, scientists published their findings: On the octogonal structure of the Nuclear Pore Complex. (146)

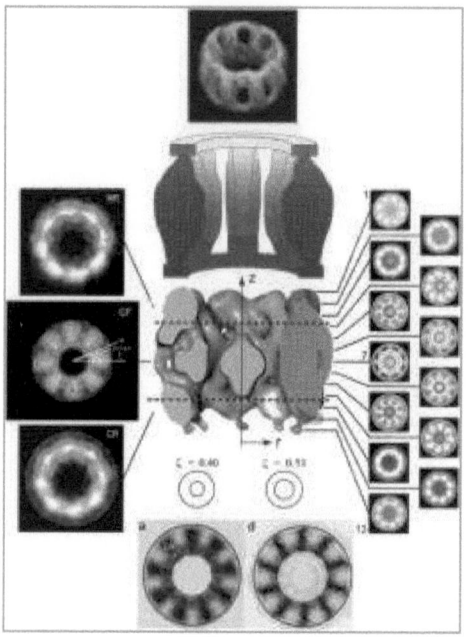

This graph is taken from the study and shows cells in rhythm with life. Cells breathe, they move, they bend, they stretch and they react to external influences. And yet they all maintain their basic life-supporting octogonal shape. Scientists concluded:

"The basic structure of the Nuclear Pore Complex (NPC) consists of an octogonal symmetry that is maintained throughout all organisms, from yeast to humans. The eightfold symmetry is most efficient to maximize the flexural stiffness and stability of each of the eight large NPC spokes.

The UVB effect in an octogonal Blu Room architecture continuously stimulates each cell to return to or maintain the life-giving octogonal basic shape.

Blu Room supports all cells in upholding or regaining their constructive form. Why is this important? Because it is the pattern of life.

The Blu Room is covered with mirror-like material from side to side, from bottom to top, from one corner to the other.

This work of art, a combination of breathtaking architecture, excellent acoustics and unique mirroring, forms the body of sound with its range of tone and color.

Floating on invisible sound waves

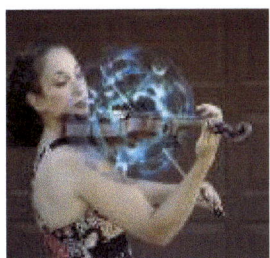

The original expression of the universe is vibration, rhythm and sound. Our whole structure, our ethereal bodies, our physiological and subatomic form, everything is permeated by vibration.

Source: www.energyfanatics.com

One of the most respected sound healers in the world today, Tom Kenyon, speaks of "strengthening in the sense of a restoration that nurtures to the depths and provides with invigorating energies. With healing sounds we can find new strength in the face of personal and global challenges. The harmonious architecture of the tunes aligns the innermost cell matrix with life's original frequency". (147)

Solfeggio-Frequencies

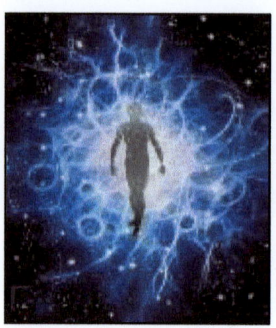 Solfeggio frequencies make up the ancient 6-tone scale thought to have been used in sacred music, including the beautiful and well known Gregorian Chants. The chants and their special tones were believed to impart spiritual blessings when sung in harmony. Each Solfeggio tone is comprised of a frequency required to balance your energy and keep your body, mind and spirit in perfect harmony. Solfeggio frequencies can also positively influence and repair our DNA.

Udo Pelkowski describes compositions in Solfeggio frequencies as music that brings us to tears, that reconnects us with our original source. (148)

All Solfeggio-frequencies lead to 3 – 6 – 9

174 Hz being connected	Digit sum 3
285 Hz Universal knowledge	Digit sum 6
396 Hz liberating guilt and fear	Digit sum 9
417 Hz Resonance, facilitating chance	Digit sum 3
528 Hz Transformation and DNA repair	Digit sum 6
639 Hz connecting/Relationships	Digit sum 9
741 Hz Expression/ Solutions	Digit sum 3
852 Hz unconditional Love	Digit sum 6
963 Hz God-Man, God-Woman	Digit sum 9

The 3, 6, and 9 are the fundamental roots of the Solfeggio frequencies.

Modern molecular biology uses 528 Hz to repair damaged DNA strands. Only when the cell membrane is responsive are repairs or reprogramming of the DNA possible. Dr. Horowitz writes in his bestselling book *Healing Codes for the Biological Apocalypse* (149) about his experiences with the frequency 528 Hz and confirms: "Solfeggio frequencies stimulate the opening of the cell for DNA re-programming". (150)

The natural tones permeate all the way to the cellular awareness. They stimulate millions of cells to 'dance' (noticeable tingling). The DNA and each individual cell adopt the state of highest order and rearrange anew. This is equivalent to a computer reset or stasis. It reminds them of their original and harmonious vibrational structures and encourages them to reorganize. Energetic blocks, chronic tensions of muscles and tissues and sometimes also 'numb spots' in the body like old injuries, scars can be addressed, loosened and often also dissolved. This is done through the law of resonance by means of vibrations and oscillations.

> *The patent document states:*
> *"As used herein, the term 'light resonance' refers to the application of light of sufficient energy to a human user to synch, encourage, or amplify resonant energy frequencies with the user's body; light resonance is believed to promote healing and well-being in human users." (183)*

These processes are controlled by the body's own brain waves.

Brainwaves – optimally structured

The human brain consists of billions of billions of neurons. They in turn are powered and nourished by billions of glial cells. Each individual nerve cell is connected to other nerve cells by thousands of branches through synapses. Together, these form a huge neuronal network: our brain - or more precisely: the central nervous system.

"The brain is clearly the most essential element for a person to unfold his full potential."
Ramtha (176)

The neurons exchange electrochemical impulses with each other and throughout the entire central nervous system of the body. Each of these electrochemical discharges generates an electromagnetic field in the form of waves. Brain waves are more far-reaching than we can describe through language. They reflect different aspects depending on where they occur in the brain, what they stimulate, what they cause and where they originate.

Five wave patterns define different states of consciousness:

Beta-waves 14 - 30 Hz
Awake, attentive, concentrated, also associated with worry, anxieties and various other forms of stress.

Alpha-waves 8 - 13 Hz
Mentally awake and yet relaxed, bridge between outer world (beta waves) and inner world (theta waves). With eyes closed, they produce a calm and pleasant feeling, the 'alpha state' or 'flow'. In the alpha state neurotransmitters are released that are essential for happiness and joy. (151)

Theta-waves 4 – 7 Hz

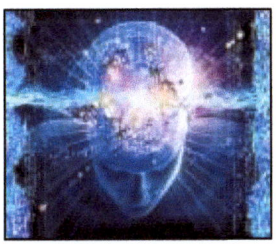 Theta - dream state, active subconscious, meditative state. Spontaneous solutions to a problem that has been pondered over for several days mostly come from the theta area. (152). The theta state causes behavioral changes and the reprogramming of negative beliefs. This in turn enables a living organism to activate the body's own self-healing. Dr. Budzynski confirms on the basis of his numerous experiences that "repair orders and reprogramming in the theta state proceed directly into the subconscious. Here they are accepted as truth. The resulting DNA changes have a lasting effect." (153) Many visitors of the Blu Room are - without consciously perceiving it - in the Theta state.

Delta-waves 0,5 – 3,5 HZ

Deep, dreamless sleep. Delta waves regulate glands and hormones. They regenerate the cells and are the source of empathy. This state triggers the healing of body and mind. The delta area also functions as the sixth sense.

Gamma-waves 30 – 70 Hz

Peak mental performance. It originates in the thalamus and traverses the front of the brain before returning. (154) Gamma waves are associated with universal and unconditional love.

> The law of vibration, a natural law proclaimed thousands of years ago by the ancient Egyptian masters, says: "Nothing rests; everything moves; everything is in motion, swings. The lower the vibration, the slower it is; the higher it is, the faster it is." (177)

Researchers at the Neurofeedback Institute confirm: "Every human being can develop his full potential when his brain waves are optimally structured and the central nervous system is balanced. An optimally functioning human brain with a stable nervous system always produces a very specific brain wave pattern that easily adapts to different states of consciousness". (155)

Vitamin D – key and lock

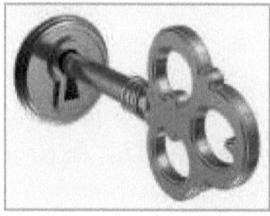

Vitamin D plays a key role in health. As the only vitamin produced by the body itself, it is involved in all vital processes. The invisible UVB component of sunlight, with a wavelength of 290-315 nanometers, is responsible for the formation of vitamin D in the skin. This corresponds to the narrow-band frequency of the UVB tubes in the Blu Room.

A 20-minute Blu Room session with 3 minutes of UVB irradiation provides a fair-skinned person with an equivalent of approximately 10,000 I.E. of orally taken vitamin D. A person with tanned or highly pigmented skin will have the benefit of about 5,000 I.E.

> A 20-minute Blu Room session with 6 minutes of UVB irradiation provides a fair-skinned person with an equivalent of approximately 20,000 I.E. of orally taken Vitamin D. A person with tanned or highly pigmented skin will have the benefit of about 10,000 I.E.

This process is controlled exclusively by the body's own DNA. The vitamin D generated is therefore DNA frequency-specific according to the special genetic code of the person. It is endogenous. Neither additional enzymatic processes nor complex synthesis steps are required. There are also no conversion losses, no transportation difficulties, no cognitive disturbances and no occupied receptors.

This is of fundamental importance because every cell needs vitamin D to control its intercellular processes.
Whether we are healthy or go through pathological processes depends among other things on an adequate vitamin D status. If we look at vitamin D as a sun hormone, every disease appears as a light-metabolism

disorder. It is not really vitamin D that the body needs, but the photons stored in vitamin D with their light properties.

Vitamin D is the door opener for:
- Thought processes, vivid creativity
- Overcoming depression and trauma
- Active immune protection against known and unknown offenders
- Strong cardiovascular system
- Cancer protection - regular cell division
- Bone and muscle building, stability, mobility
- Pancreas, blood sugar regulation
- Mental development and longevity,
- Telomere extension
- Stem cell growth, the future in general

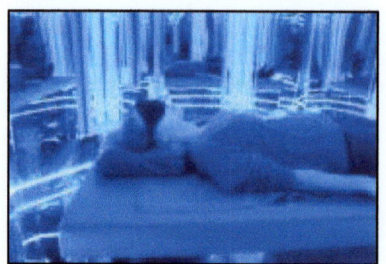

What happens in this composition of sacred geometry, mirror, light, sound and frequency, shielded from external influences?

The visitor lies in the heart of this room. After just a few minutes with UVB light, all 700 billion cells are flooded with photons. Microtubules, the light transport channels, ensure that the brain and body receive coherent light. An active vitamin D production begins. (156)

The whole body breathes in this atmosphere of light. All body fluids are also subject to this dynamic energy and structure themselves.
The blood vessels with their finest branches, the lymph, all intra- and extracellular tissues and all water molecules are affected.
In March 2018, researchers discovered a complicated fluid-filled channeling system in the deep connective tissue beneath the surface of the skin. (157) They also found these fascinating canal systems in the lining of the lungs, digestive tract and urinary tract. Under UVB light, a vibrating and honeycomb-shaped intermediate medium or exclusion zone discovered by Pollack develops in all these body fluids. (158)
As the structured liquid crystal zone increases, it expels troubling substances just as a growing glacier does with rocks.

Order is created. In this state of deep relaxation, the circulation of all liquid substances in the body improves. Slags and toxins are excreted and good nutrients for construction and repair are inserted. This dynamic is invigorating and regenerative, even unlimited.

If we scrutinize the bridge medium, we find that all individually shaped systems such as DNA, nervous, immune and metabolic systems will also change. Therefore the order factor is in effect. Coherence is established.

Self-healing impulses trigger immediate change. New perspectives emerge, telomeres grow and stem cells flood into diseased systems. A state of stasis develops, comparable to a 'reset' on the computer. Tensions in the Yin Yang body collapse and we become one.

The entrance to deeper soul levels and extended states of consciousness open up.

Deep harmony characterizes these Blu Room moments. Neither past nor future - just NOW.

In a healthy body, 10 million cells die second after second and 10 million new cells are created.

In a three-minute Blu Room session, 180 billion cells are developed in this tension-free state with an optimal life matrix.

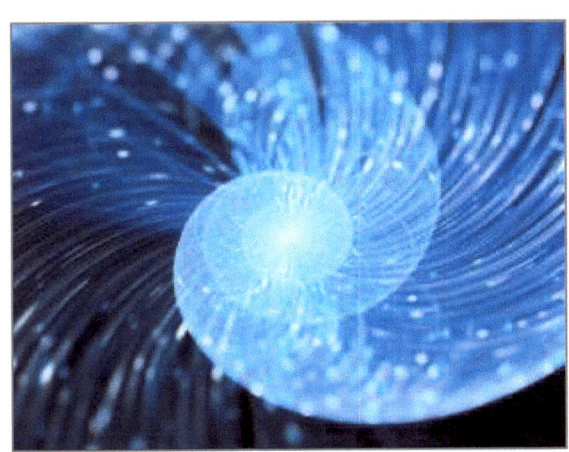

In deep relaxation it is easy for us to maintain control over the thoughts that occupy our mind. We decide freely which thoughts we want to nourish and which one we want to dispense with. We begin by using the power of thoughts for a better life.

"Faster than every 1/40th of a second, the microtubules of neural cells fluctuate in and our geometric resonance, creating our physical space (body/mind) to align (harmonically) with nonlocal singularity – giving us a picture of the microtubule's geometry, our quantum consciousness" says research scientist Lindsay Briner, (159)

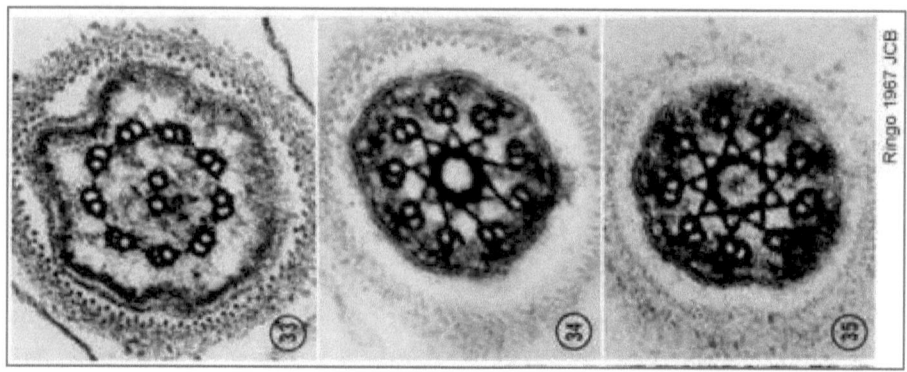

How fast is 1/40 of a second? So fast that we can't process it. This means that our subconscious mind moves so fast to judge and understand our environment and make decisions in our body before our frontal lobe is aware of it.

40 times a second, it has an effect on our physiology. If we are depressed, we don't like yourself, we don't like your job, we are negative, we are happy – our microtubules respond.

The Blu Room stops our programs, resets and allows a new single signal to act. Harmony!

The Blu Room also has an effect without our intervention, our thinking, our analyzing, our special effort and cooperation.

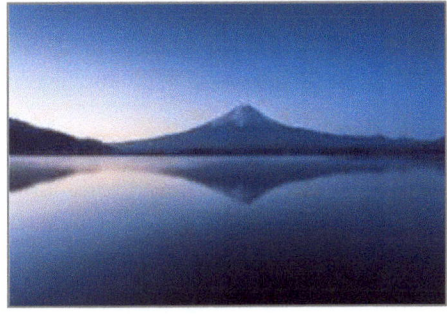

Dr. Martinez is convinced that "New and authentic ideas do not come through thinking, but through access into deep sources".

- Deep relaxation
- faster healing processes
- Relieving mental stress and anxiety.
- Improved health and quality of life
- Significant increase in vitamin D3 levels in blood serum
- Deeper focus and concentration
- Increased creativity and problem solving
- self-perception
- self-confidence, self-respect, self-love

Prof. Dr. Popp explains the phenomenon of the Blu Room in his own way: "We have to understand how something builds up in the inter-action of matter and electromagnetic field that can be attributed the property of coherence. Coherence means that there is the ability to perform an interaction in which each part can communicate with each other." (160)

Nobel Laureate Dr. Hans-Peter Dürr says:
"Not everything can be proven. Some things have to be experienced.
It is a venture to explore the unknown." (184)

Blu Room users report a wide range of experiences after their visit to the Blu Room:

Unrivalled - the reports are individual

We humans are unique beings. Each of us begins his or her life with his very own code, his own blueprint, the DNA. So all experiences in the Blu Room are individual.
This is exactly what numerous experiences of Blu Room visitors reflect.

Saved 300.000 Dollars with the right idea
In a single Blu Room session the businessman Gerald recognized the only financial solution for his case, saving him a small fortune. (Blu Room, Soazza)

In spite of all the know-it-alls
42 year old Sabine is finally pregnant. (Blu Room, Olympia)

Carlos wanted to know
Before the European Championship he visited the Blu Room. He was jumping his highest. (Blu Room, Weimar)

The weight decreased, the self-esteem scale increased
Julia, 135 kg, very low self-esteem. Before starting a diet, she visited the Blu Room 3 times a week for 4 weeks. After that time, she laughed again, felt more self-esteem and was able to lose weight without any stress. (Blu Room, Olympia)

Leonie did it
Leonie was a genius, yet had terrible exam anxiety. Before the final exam she visited the Blu Room. Focused and calm she wrote the exam and passed. (Blu Room, Olympia)

Depressed after delivery
Elisa delivered her first born son, yet suffered from childbed depression. Elisa visited the Blu Room twice a week. Soon her joy returned and her hormones were balanced. (Blu Room, Vienna)

As an autist out of the "pigeonhole"
Carlo, who at the age of eight had already been put in a "pigeonhole" as an autist as far as education was concerned. He was visiting the Blu Room for several weeks. In school he began to show higher cognitive awareness and at home he argued with his siblings. (Blu Room, Weimar)

A drive of 1,000 miles driven - and it was worth it
Steve came to the Blu Room because he was struggling with diseases. After the first Blu Room visit he realized that the illnesses were the result of his own negative attitudes. Blu Room visits helped to overcome deep emotional and spiritual blockages. "I now have peace in areas of my life where there used to be a lot of fear and stress. I drove 1,000 miles to get here. It was worth it." (Blu Room, Wellness Center Washington MO)

Bone marrow cancer in remission with Blu Room treatment
In 1990, Nikki Bertone was diagnosed with multiple myeloma (plasmocytoma, bone marrow cancer). After 6 years with strict treatment regimen and chemotherapy, the cancer began to spread again in January 2016. Blood analysis before and after treatments showed impressive improvements. The cancer markers returned to normal after further Blu Room visits. (161)

Vertebral body restored after osteochondritis
In 2014, a physician was diagnosed with erosive osteochondritis on the basis of an MRI. He began regular Blu Room visits in March 2016. An MRI performed in June 2016 including PET/CT showed "complete healing of erosive osteochondritis". (162) (Blu Room, Bad Mergentheim)

Progressive heart failure after Blu Room visits suspended
In June 2011, Yumo experienced severe chest pain after a football match. The diagnosis was a blockage of the coronary artery. In February 2017, after Blu Room visits, Yumo received the latest test results. The EEG and heart function level were normal. (163) (Blu Room, Japan)

I'm old enough now
Blu Room Muelheim reports of a 12 year old girl. 2 years ago during a school swimming lesson she had a traumatic experience with her swimming teacher. Since then she never went swimming again and she always needed her mother.
After the 5th Blu Room session she wanted to go to the swimming pool with her mother. And in the Blu Room, she went by herself now. "I'm old enough to go in there alone now." (Blu Room Muelheim 2017)

Fit again for the mountains after Parkinson's disease
His typical symptoms were muscle tremor and slower movements. He took his medication and frequently visited the Blu Room in Lugano. 12 months later he was able to resume his beloved mountain hikes. (Blu Room Stella del Nord, 2017)

Flexible pupils make night driving possible again
Carola, 52 years old, has suffered from rigid pupils for years. Due to the lack of response to light stimuli, night vision was severely impaired. This prevented her driving the car in the dark. She went to the Blu Room twice a week for three weeks. Slowly the pupils became more flexible. Today she is safely driving at night. (Blu Room Salamander, 2017)

Hyperthyroidism finally dismissed
In July 2015, a type of hyperthyroidism called Graves disease (Graves' disease) was diagnosed. With conventional medications, the symptoms were partially under control, but she was not cured. After several Blu Room visits, blood tests showed normal thyroid function. It is now 1 ½ years after healing without any relapse of the disease. (164)

Happy inside and out - without tormenting eczema
A seborrheic eczema has been plaguing Diana for 20 years. Apart from the fact that she felt ugly, it was also very painful. After some Blu Room visits the situation became much better, the intense pain and burning sensation was almost gone. After three weeks the skin was back to normal. (Blu Room, Boffalora Wellness Center 2017)

Chronic wound healed
Pat, 77 years old, fell and tore open the skin of her right lower leg, resulting in a 5 cm open cut. The wound did not heal for months despite dressings and external treatment. After some Blu Room visits the wound was completely closed. (165) (Blu Room, Wellness Center Washington, MO 2018)

Severe diarrhea in calves treated
A farmer visited the Blu Room because of his own physical problems. He incidentally mentioned that he had problems with his pregnant cows and calves. There were many miscarriages and the newborn calves often suffered from severe diarrhea. Since he used the Blu Room himself, we recommended that he take some Blu Room water home for his animals. He took this advice to heart and regularly gave the calves and pregnant cows Blu Room water. Already after six weeks he reported enthusiastically that the problems had disappeared. (166) (Blu Room BluRelax, 2017)

Elliot, the small dog is no longer afraid of thunderstorms
I have a two-year-old dog named Elliot. When I found out that animals were also allowed in the Blu Room, I really wanted to try it out. I was curious what would change. To my surprise, something happened that I never expected.

Elliot is afraid of thunderstorms. He runs back and forth, can't rest for hours, pants strongly and can't be distracted with treats. Three days after our visit to the Blu Room there was a violent thunderstorm and Elliot just lay relaxed on his blanket. (Blu Room, Blaue Pause, 2018)

Tension gone, the muscles relaxed and the breathing is freely
I had been having a slight muscular tension between my shoulder blades for several weeks. When I lay down on the couch in the Blu Room, after a few seconds I began to feel an acute discomfort between my shoulder blades where the tension was. I began to think the couch was too hard, and wondered how I was going to put up with this distracting pain for the duration of the treatment.

For the next 15-20 seconds the pain got steadily worse. Then I felt a sensation as if someone were pulling in opposite directions on my spine between my shoulder blades, and the pain got worse. Suddenly I heard a loud "pop" sound from where the pain was. Instantly everything relaxed in my back and all traces of the pain disappeared immediately.

During all this time I was lying totally relaxed on my back, despite the pain, and was exerting no force whatever in any direction. What was even more exciting is that when I was returning down the hallway to the Arena, I realized that my whole breathing pattern had changed. I was now taking deep breaths without effort, about twice what had been normal for me before. (Blu Room Yelm)

The third session was the absolute game changer for me.
Jacqueline Molina's Story
Being a skeptic towards everything from the medical field to the paranormal.

Since the age of 11, I have had brutally painful menstrual cramps that continued throughout my entire life. I have tried almost every natural supplement/vitamin for so many years without ever having significant relief if any.

Furthermore, with my work being extremely physical, throughout 17 years I have sustained multiple injuries including herniated discs, pinched nerves, severe osteoarthritis and stenosis through discovery from CT scans, MRI, x-rays, and neurologist. I underwent many therapies.

A friend told me about the Blu Room. I slept quite well that night after the first session. I gave it another shot and went for a second session. This time I felt calmness but nothing too remarkable. The third session was the absolute game changer for me. My back pain was diminished tremendously. I decided to go once a week after that. The following menstrual cycle was easy, tolerable. The second was even easier, and by the third I had no pain whatsoever, no PMS either.

Not only did the Blu Room sessions help with my pain, which was my main reason for trying it, it has helped me be more focused, have better deeper restful sleep, have a sense of wellbeing, clearer thoughts and an ability to let certain things go from the past that we may be clinging to and don't realize it. (Blu Room Univers Bleu, Canada)

A good night's sleep again

"From my early age I always had trouble waking up in the morning. I often had so many dreams at night and woke up feeling tired. Also, I have been under stress as I have had to work hard to catch up with classes at school. After my second session, I woke up easily after a good night's sleep and even feel refreshed. I keep going to the Blu Room on a regular basis". (Blu Room Japan)

This special testimonial moves:

Dayle fought as a US soldier in the Vietnam War that lasted two decades. The brutality of the war could hardly be surpassed. He returned physically alive from the war zone, but with severe psychological wounds. Back in the U.S.A., he was unable to find his place in life again. At night he dreamed of war and cruelty. He lost his job and his family broke apart. He fell into a deep depression with suicidal intentions. No pill helped him. So he came to Dr. Martinez, Absolute Health Clinic, Olympia, WA. The doctor offered him to visit the Blu Room as often as he wanted. After many visits, he enjoys life again.

> A few months ago an interviewer asked him: "What did you get out of the Blu Room? Dayle replied: "The Blu Room is a gift". The journalist wasn't satisfied with that. "Did the Blu Room bring you hope?" "I went to war with hope of peace. I'm bitterly disappointed," Dayle replies. "Did the Blu Room give you a new life?" "No, I lived before too, just every night with the nightmares. In the morning I woke up and life went on with the same pictures buzzing in my mind's eye - Blu Room gave me a perspective. Blu Room showed me that I have really strong skills. I got a new job. Blu Room gave me self-love and the appreciation for life again. The pictures of the war are still coming, but they don't concern me anymore. Now I live with my family again. (143)

Bathing in Light

The patent paper documents:
„The terms "bathe" or "bathing" as used herein in conjunction with a light therapy according to the invention refers to concentrating light in a three-dimensional space to surround, or partially surround, a human user. Because light travels both as a wave and as a particle, a space with a measurable presence of light waves and particles may be said to have a light density. The greater the light density in a given three-dimensional space around a human user, and the more that the light density surrounds the human user, the more the user, and any other object within the three-dimensional space, may be said to be "bathed" in the light.." (183)

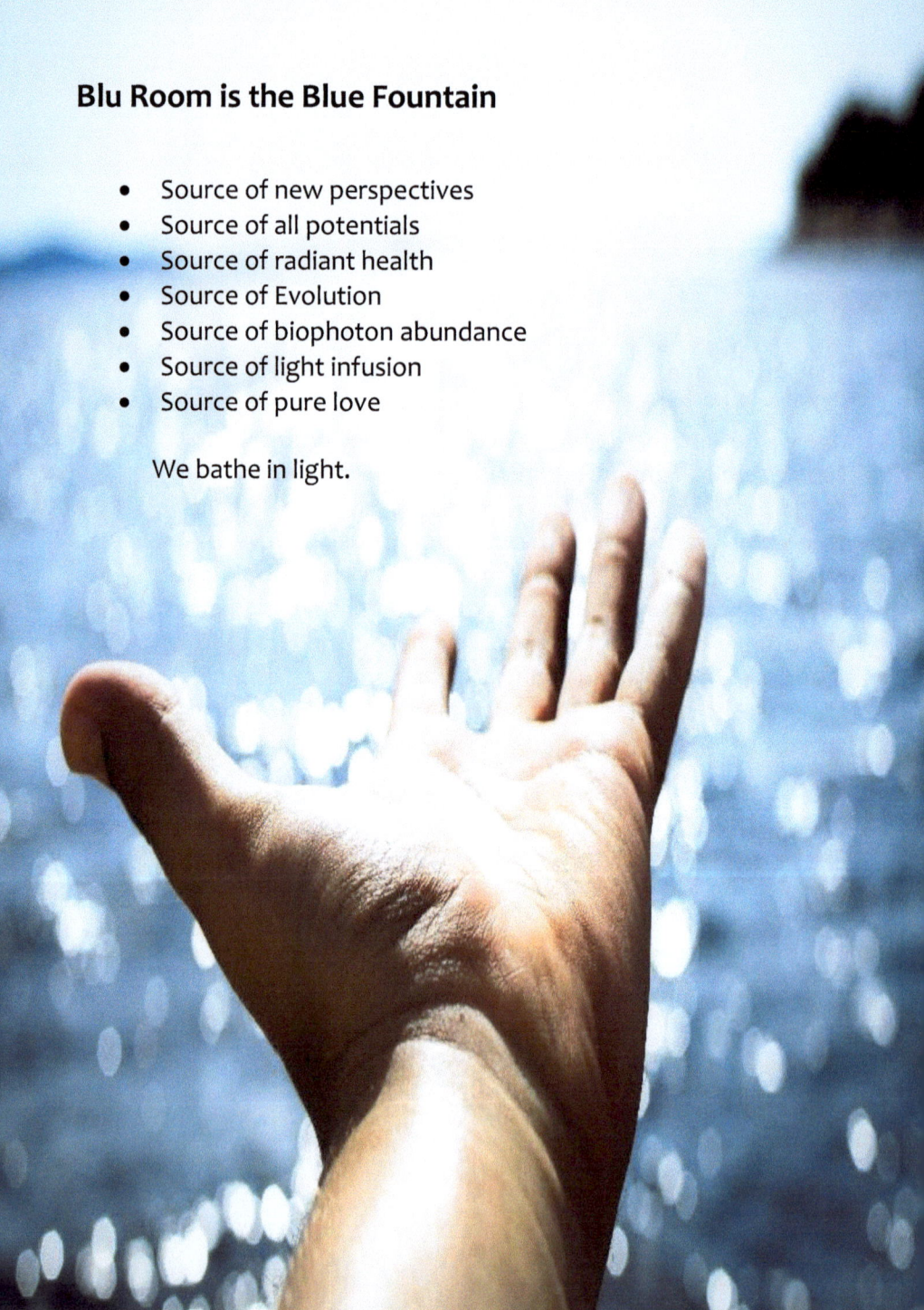

Blu Room is the Blue Fountain

- Source of new perspectives
- Source of all potentials
- Source of radiant health
- Source of Evolution
- Source of biophoton abundance
- Source of light infusion
- Source of pure love

We bathe in light.

Bathing in light is a special experience for the body, soul and spirit. It gives deep relaxation, self-awareness and wholeness.

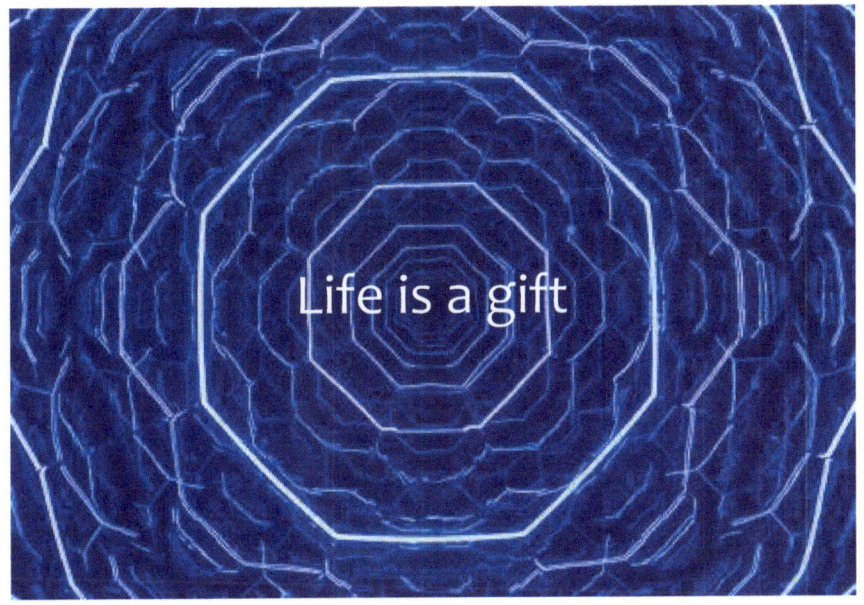

Blu Room is the future of medicine and personal well-being.
Blu Room affects you physically, mentally and spiritually.
Blu Room puts you back in charge of your life.

The Author

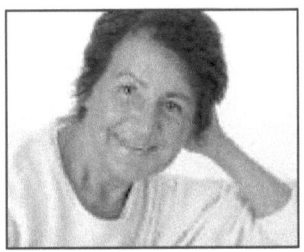

For many years, Irmgard Maria Gräf has been investigating important life factors with her heart and analytical mind. She passionately explores solutions in the visible world, nature and in the invisible world of quantum physics. Her work is characterized by many experiences during a long stay in the U.S.A. Conversations with indigenous Indians, visionary astronauts, ingenious inventors, masters of ancient wisdom and advanced medical therapists inspired her.

University of Alabama in Huntsville, U.S.A;
RFA Germany, , RSE, WA U.S.A.; Dr. Budwig Academy; Institute Vitamin Delta, many advanced and further training courses in the field of naturopathy and applied quantum physics.

Publications:
- *Die Quark-Öl-Kur – Die Heilwirkungen der Öl-Eiweiß-Kost nach Dr. Budwig*, ViaNova Verlag 2014 (167)
- *Mein Blut ein Weg zu mir – was mein Blut mir sagt* , Michaels Verlag 2014 (168)
- *Blu Room –Experience the future. Building bridges with light, frequency and sound* (2017) (169)
- *Blu Room – Zukunft hautnah erleben* (2017) (34)
- *Die Blaue Quelle – Theorie und Potenzial der Blu Room Technologie* (2018) (170)

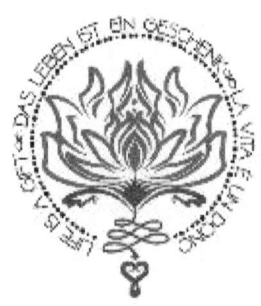

The Blu Room does not replace any medical therapy, however the effect in the Blu Room can support or accelerate conventional medical as well as naturopathic therapies.

You will find detailed reports with references in the master book: *Blu Room - Experience the future* (169), and on the websites: www.bluroom.com, www.bluroom-dasbuch.com, or the respective websites of the Blu Room operators.

Blu Rooms can be found in the Argentina, Austria, Canada, Colombia, Ecuador, Germany, Italy, Japan, Mexico, Switzerland, Taiwan and the United States of America.

The exact locations can be found at:
www.bluroom.com/pages/locations.aspx.

For more information about the Blu Room, contact: Blu Room Enterprises, LLC, P.O. Box 5895, Lacey, WA
98509, USA. www.bluroom.com

Sources of photo material and graphics

Own archive
123 rf stockfoto https://de.123rf.com
Fotolia https://www.fotolia.com
Dreamstime https://de.dreamstime.com/
Anton Blättler, Lukas, Hannah Nelson, Abhiram Prakash,
Doris Lippuner.
Graphik: Heidi Schupfner, Marion Collenberg
Other sources are documented

References:

1. Gräf, Irmgard Maria. *Blu Room - Zukunft hautnah erleben. Mit Licht Frequenz und Klang Brücken bauen.* Maienfeld : s.n., 2017. ISBN 978-3-00-058322-3.

2. Pfleiderer, Heinrich , Alfred RüttenauerWolfgang Petzold. https://link.springer.com/chapter/10.1007%2F978-3-642-50693-2_10. [Online]

3. Ingold, Niklaus. *Lichtduschen: Geschichte einer Gesundheitstechnik.* 2015. 978-3034012768.

4. Wolff, Ori. *NetzwerkMensch.* Berlin : LehmannMedia, 2017. ISBN 978-3-38541-703-9.

5. Popp, Prof. Dr. F.A. *Biophotonen- Neue Horizonte in der Medizin. Von den Grundlagen zur Biophoton 2006.* 2006. ISBN-10: 3830472676.

6. https://www.universitystudy.ca/canadian-universities/ryerson-university/. [Online]

7. Bludorf, Franz, Fosar, Grazyna. *Vernetzte Intelligenz: Die Natur geht online - Gruppenbewusstsein, Genetik, Gravitation.* s.l. : Omega Verlag Bongart-Meier, 2001. 978-3930243235.

8. Shuttler, Lance. The Mind Unleashed. *New Science: DNA begins as a quantum wave.* [Online] Jan 2017. https://themindunleashed.com/2017/01/new-science-dna-begins-quantum-wave.html.

9. Rudolph, Denis. https://www.frustfrei-lernen.de/biologie/genotyp-phaenotyp-unterschied.html. [Online] Dez 28, 2017.

10. Ogilvie, Jennifer. https://www.upi.com/Science_News/2018/03/20/Researchers-capture-image-of-first-step-of-photosynthesis/7571521568294/. [Online] 2018.

11. Maseeh, Rathish Nair and Arun. https://www.ncbi.nlm.nih.gov/pmc/articles/PMC3356951/. *Vitamin D: The "sunshine" vitamin.* [Online] 2012.

12. Holick, Michael F., Neil C. Binkley, Heike A. Bischoff-Ferrari, Catherine M. Gordon, David A. Hanley, Robert P. Heaney, M. Hassan Murad, and Connie M. Weaver. Evaluation, treatment, and prevention of vitamin D deficiency: an Endocrine Society clinical practice guideline. *PubMed.* [Online] 2011. https://www.ncbi.nlm.nih.gov/pubmed/21646368.

13. Silvagno F1, De Vivo E, Attanasio A, Gallo V, Mazzucco G, Pescarmona G. Mitochondrial localization of vitamin D receptor in human platelets and differentiated megakaryocytes. *PubMed.* [Online] Jan 2010. https://www.ncbi.nlm.nih.gov/pubmed/20107497.

14. Yanping Lin, a John L. Ubels,b Mark P. Schotanus,b Zhaohong Yin,c Victorina Pintea,c Bruce D. Hammock,a and Mitchell A. Watskyc. Enhancement of Vitamin D Metabolites in the Eye following Vitamin D3 Supplementation and UV-B Irradiation. *PMC.* [Online] Oct 2013. https://www.ncbi.nlm.nih.gov/pmc/articles/PMC3572765/.

15. *Grant WB. The prevalence of multiple sclerosis in 3 US communities: the role of vitamin D. Prev Chronic Dis. 2010;7:A89–, author reply A90.* https://www.ncbi.nlm.nih.gov/pmc/articles/PMC3897598/ : s.n.

16. Immunology, and Allergy Clinics of North America. Science Direct. *http://www.sciencedirect.com/science/article/pii/S0889856110000433.* [Online] Aug 2010.

17. Bhalla AK, Amento EP, Clemens TL, Holick MF, Krane SM. Specific high-affinity receptors for 1,25-dihydroxyvitamin D3 in human peripheral blood mononuclear cells:

presence in monocytes and induction in T lymphocytes following activation. J Clin Endocrinol . *PubMed.* [Online] 1983. https://www.ncbi.nlm.nih.gov/pubmed/6313738.
18. *https://www.ncbi.nlm.nih.gov/pmc/articles/PMC3897598/.*
19. *Wacker M, Holick MF. Vitamin D - effects on skeletal and extraskeletal health and the need for supplementation. Nutrients. 2013;5:111–48. doi: 10.3390/nu5010111.* https://www.ncbi.nlm.nih.gov/pmc/articles/PMC3897598/ : s.n.
20. Adams JS, Gacad MA. Characterization of 1 alpha-hydroxylation of vitamin D3 sterols by cultured alveolar macrophages from patients with sarcoidosis. J Exp Med. *PubMed.* [Online] 1985. https://www.ncbi.nlm.nih.gov/pubmed/3838552.
21. *Schultz M, Butt AG. Is the north to south gradient in inflammatory bowel disease a global phenomenon? Expert Rev Gastroenterol Hepatol. 2012;6:445–7. doi: 10.1586/egh.12.31.* https://www.ncbi.nlm.nih.gov/pmc/articles/PMC3897598/ : s.n.
22. Sean T. Corbetta, Oya Hillb, Ajay K. Nangiaa, , . Vitamin D receptor found in human sperm. *Science Direct.* [Online] Dec 2006.
http://www.sciencedirect.com/science/article/pii/S0090429506021339.
23. Baker AR, McDonnell DP, Hughes M, et al. Cloning and expression of full-length cDNA encoding human vitamin D receptor. Proc Natl Acad Sci U S A. . *PubMed.* [Online] 1988. https://www.ncbi.nlm.nih.gov/pubmed/2835767.
24. *Grant WB. Ecological studies of the UVB-vitamin D-cancer hypothesis. Anticancer Res.* 2012;32:223–36. https://www.ncbi.nlm.nih.gov/pmc/articles/PMC3897598/ : s.n.
25. Shaffer PL1, Gewirth DT. Vitamin D receptor-DNA interactions. *PubMed.* [Online] https://www.ncbi.nlm.nih.gov/pubmed/15193458.
26. Queen Mary University of London.
http://www.qmul.ac.uk/media/news/items/smd/180791.html. [Online] Sep 2016.
27. Cannell JJ1, Vieth R, Umhau JC, Holick MF, Grant WB, Madronich S, Garland CF, Giovannucci E. Epidemic influenza and vitamin D. *PubMed.* [Online] Dec 2006. https://www.ncbi.nlm.nih.gov/pubmed/16959053.
28. Edlich RF, Mason SS, Dahlstrom JJ, Swainston E, Long WB 3rd, Gubler K. Pandemic preparedness for swine flu influenza in the United States. *PubMed.* [Online] 2009. https://www.ncbi.nlm.nih.gov/pubmed/20102323.
29. Torres, Marco. Vitamin D Proven More Effective Than Both Anti-Viral Drugs and Vaccines At Preventing The Flu. *PreventDisease.* [Online] Oct 2013.
https://preventdisease.com/news/13/102213_Vitamin-D-Proven-More-Effective-Anti-Viral-Drugs-Vaccines-Preventing-Flu.shtml.
30. Canell, JJ, et al. Randomized trial of vitamin D supplementation to prevent seasonal influenza A in schoolchildren1,2,3. *The American Journal of Clinical Nutrition.* [Online] 2010. http://ajcn.nutrition.org/content/91/5/1255.full.
31. https://www.uni-muenchen.de/informationen_fuer/presse/presseinformationen/2011/f-30-11.html. [Online] 2011.
32. Entzündliche Hauterkrankungen. *Medizinische Fakultät Universität München.* [Online] 2010. http://www.med.uni-muenchen.de/forschung/schwerpunkte/infektion/artikel_entzuendlichehaut/index.html.

33. *Morimoto S, Yoshikawa K, Kozuka T et al: An open study of vitamin D3 treatment in psoriasis vulgaris. Br J Dermatol; 115(4):421-429. 1986.*
34. Gräf, Irmgard Maria. *Blu Room - Zukunft hautnah erleben. Mit Licht Frequenz und Klang Brücken bauen.* Maienfeld : s.n., 2017. ISBN 978-3-00-058322-3.
35. Reichrath, Jörg (Ed.). *http://www.springer.com/us/book/9781493904365.* s.l. : Springer, 2014. ISBN 978-1-4939-0437-2.
36. Helden, Raimund von, MD. Was können wir gegen Strahlenschäden tun? Vitamin D als natürliches Zellschutz-System ! *Vitamin D Service.* [Online] 2016. https://www.vitamindservice.de/was-k%C3%B6nnen-wir-gegen-strahlensch%C3%A4den-tun-vitamin-d-als-nat%C3%BCrliches-zellschutz-system.
37. Lohr, Aaron. Chemical Exposure Linked to Lower Vitamin D Levels. *Endocrine Society.* [Online] Sep 20, 2016.
38. Was ist BPA und wo steckt es drin? *Global 2000.* [Online] https://www.global2000.at/was-ist-bpa-und-wo-steckt-es-drin.
39. Lüscher, Dr. Heinz. Vitamin D. *Praxis für Vitalstoffmedizin.* [Online] https://www.vitalstoffmedizin.ch/index.php/de/38-vitalstoffmedizin.
40. Hallelder, Günter, Wolfgang Simon, Viktor von Toenges. Neurowissen - Multiple Sklerose - Entstehung und kausale Beahndlung. [Online] 2012. http://www.myoreflex.de/media/downloads/Mosetter_Neurowissen_10_.pdf.
41. Rolle von Vitamin D bei allergischen Erkrankungen – eine Standortbestimmung. *Journal MED.* [Online] Feb 01, 2016. https://www.journalmed.de/schwerpunkte/anzeigen/Vitamin_D_allergische_Erkrankunge n_Standortbestimmung.
42. Hoogendijk WJ1, Lips P, Dik MG, Deeg DJ, Beekman AT, Penninx BW. Depression is associated with decreased 25-hydroxyvitamin D and increased parathyroid hormone levels in older adults. *PubMed.* [Online] May 2008. https://www.ncbi.nlm.nih.gov/pubmed/18458202.
43. Bertone-Johnson . Vitamin D and the occurrence of depression: causal association or circumstantial evidence? *PubMed.* [Online] Aug 2009. https://www.ncbi.nlm.nih.gov/pubmed/19674344.
44. Vaziri F1, Nasiri S2, Tavana Z3, Dabbaghmanesh MH4, Sharif F5, Jafari P6. Perinatal depression decreased 40 percent with just a few weeks of 2,000 IU of vitamin D – RCT Aug 2016. *VitaminDWiki.* [Online] Aug 20, 2016. http://www.vitamindwiki.com/Perinatal+depression+decreased+40+percent+with+just+a +few+weeks+of+2%2C000+IU+of+vitamin+D+%E2%80%93+RCT+Aug+2016.
45. Saad K1, Abdel-Rahman AA2, Elserogy YM2, Al-Atram AA3, El-Houfey AA4, Othman HA5, Bjørklund G6, Jia F7, Urbina MA8,9, Abo-Elela MG10, Ahmad FA1, Abd El-Baseer KA10, Ahmed AE10, Abdel-Salam AM11. Randomized controlled trial of vitamin D supplementation in children with autism spectrum disorder. *PubMed.* [Online] Nov 21, 2016. https://www.ncbi.nlm.nih.gov/pubmed/27868194.
46. Kwon KY, Jo KD, Lee MK, Oh M, Kim EN, Park J, Kim JS, Youn J, Oh E, Kim HT, Oh MY, Jang W. Low Serum Vitamin D Levels May Contribute to Gastric Dysmotility in de novo

Parkinson's Disease. *PubMed.* [Online] Jan 7, 2016.
https://www.ncbi.nlm.nih.gov/pubmed/26735311.

47. Oshiro, Rebeccca. An overview on current evidence on vitamin D and brain disorders. *Vitamin D Council.* [Online] Sep 2013. https://www.vitamindcouncil.org/an-overview-on-current-evidence-on-vitamin-d-and-brain-disorders/.

48. Worm, Dr. Nicolai. *Heilkraft Vitamin D Wie das Sonnenvitamin vor Herzinfarkt, Krebs und anderen Zivilisationskrankheiten schützt.* München : systemed, 2011.

49. Irene, Berres. Vitamin D könnte Demenzrisiko reduzieren. *Spiegel online.* [Online] Aug 07, 2014. http://www.spiegel.de/gesundheit/diagnose/alzheimer-vitamin-d-mangel-koennte-demenzrisiko-erhoehen-a-984548.html.

50. Holló,András , Zsófia Clemens, and Péter Lakatos. Epilepsy and Vitamin D. *tandfonline.* [Online] 2014. http://www.tandfonline.com/doi/abs/10.3109/00207454.2013.847836.

51. May, Epilepsy Behav. 2012 and 11., 24(1):131-3. doi: 10.1016/j.yebeh.2012.03.011. Epub 2012 Apr. Correction of vitamin D deficiency improves seizure control in epilepsy: a pilot study. *OubMed.* [Online] May 2012. https://www.ncbi.nlm.nih.gov/pubmed/22503468.

52. Goldberg, P. Multiple sclerosis: vitamin D and calcium as environmental determinants of prevalence. *Taylors Francis Online.* [Online] 1974. http://www.tandfonline.com/doi/abs/10.1080/00207237408709630.

53. ACHESON ED, BACHRACH CA, WRIGHT FM. Some comments on the relationship of the distribution of multiple sclerosis to latitude, solar radiation, and other variables. *PubMed.* [Online] 1960. https://www.ncbi.nlm.nih.gov/pubmed/13681205.

54. Schweikart, Dr. J. VITAMIN D UND MULTIPLE SKLEROSE. *Vitamin D Mangel.* [Online] http://www.vitamind.net/multiple-sklerose-ms/.

55. Fitzgerald KC1, Munger KL1, Köchert K2, Arnason BG3, Comi G4, Cook S5, Goodin DS6, Filippi M7, Hartung HP8, Jeffery DR9, O'Connor P10, Suarez G11, Sandbrink R12, Kappos L13, Pohl C14, Ascherio A15. Association of Vitamin D Levels With Multiple Sclerosis Activity and Progression in Patients Receiving Interferon Beta-1b. *PubMed.* [Online] Dec 2015. https://www.ncbi.nlm.nih.gov/pubmed/26458124.

56. Cannell, John, MD. Is it sunshine or vitamin D that helps multiple sclerosis (MS) patients? *Vitamin D Council.* [Online] Oct 16, 2015. https://www.vitamindcouncil.org/is-it-sunshine-or-vitamin-d-that-helps-multiple-sclerosis-ms-patients/.

57. Studie bestätigt Verbindung zwischen Vitamin-D-Mangel und höherem Multiple Sklerose-Risiko in Finnland. *dmsg.* [Online] Oct 17, 2016. https://www.dmsg.de/multiple-sklerose-news/ms-forschung/news-article/News/detail/studie-bestaetigt-verbindung-zwischen-vitamin-d-mangel-und-hoeherem-multiple-sklerose-risiko-in-finn/?no_cache=1&cHash=88cd9ac9b9f47ac6d8c73438869f35bb.

58. Nonnenmacher, Dr. med. Graue Substanz. *Symptomat.* [Online] Oct 2016. http://symptomat.de/Graue_Substanz.

59. Closer look: vitamin D may help protect the brain in MS patients. *vitamindcouncil.* [Online] Nov 30, 2015. ps://www.vitamindcouncil.org/closer-look-vitamin-d-may-help-protect-the-brain-in-ms-patients/.

60. Mowry EM1, Pelletier D2, Gao Z3, Howell MD3, Zamvil SS4, Waubant E4. Vitamin D in clinically isolated syndrome: evidence for possible neuroprotection. *PubMed.* [Online] Feb

2016.
https://www.ncbi.nlm.nih.gov/pubmed/?term=Vitamin+D+in+clinically+isolated+syndrom
e%3A+evidence+for+possible+neuroprotection.
61. Menning, Hans. *Das psychische Immunsystem*. Göttingen : Hogrefe Verlag, 2015. ISBN
978-3-8017-2495-5.
62. Mayo Clinic Staff. Osteoporosis. *Mayo Clinic*. [Online]
http://www.mayoclinic.org/diseases-conditions/osteoporosis/home/ovc-20207808.
63. Bouillon, Roger, Tatsuo Suda. Vitamin D: calcium and bone homeostasis during
evolution. *BoneKEyReports*. [Online] 2014.
http://www.nature.com/bonekeyreports/2014/140108/bonekey2013214/full/bonekey201321
4.html.
64. Bess Dawson-Hughes, M.D., Susan S. Harris, D.Sc., Elizabeth A. Krall, Ph.D., and Gerard
E. Dallal, Ph.D. Dawson-Hughes B, Harris SS, Krall EA, et al. Effect of calcium and vitamin D
supplementation on bone density in men and women 65 years of age or older. N Engl J
Med. 337:670-676. 1997. *The NEW ENGLAND JOURNAL of MEDICINE*. [Online] 1997.
http://www.nejm.org/doi/full/10.1056/NEJM199709043371003#t=article.
65. Bor, EJ1, van den Hoeven-van Kasteel W, Kelder JC, Lems WF. Prevalence and
correction of severe hypovitaminosis D in patients over 50 years with a low-energy
fracture. *PubMed*. [Online] Mar 2015. https://www.ncbi.nlm.nih.gov/pubmed/25852112.
66. Bowles, Jeff T. *The miraculous results of extremely high doses of the sunshine hormone
vitamine D*. Sep : CreateSpace Independent Publishing Platform; Auflage: 1 (2. September
2013), 2013. ISBN-13: 978-1491243824.
67. Ekwaru, John Paul, Jennifer D. Zwicker, Michael F. Holick, Edward Giovannucci, Paul J.
Veugelers. The Importance of Body Weight for the Dose Response Relationship of Oral
Vitamin D Supplementation and Serum 25-Hydroxyvitamin D in Healthy Volunteers.
VitaminDWiki. [Online] Nov 2014. John Paul Ekwaru, Jennifer D. Zwicker, Michael F.
Holick, Edward Giovannucci, Paul J. Veugelers.
68. Jacobo Wortsman Matsuoka Lois Y Matsuoka, L.Y Michael F J Wortsman Matsuoka,
Lois Y Jacobo, Wortsman Zhiren Lu L Matsuoka TaiC Chen Tai Michael Holick Tai C, Chen
Jacobo Lois Y Lu Zhiren Lu Holick Chen, TC Chen, Tai C Tai Chen Tai C Wortsman.
Decreased bioavailability of vitamin D in obesity1,2,3. *American Society for Clinical
Nutrition*. [Online] 2000. http://ajcn.nutrition.org/content/72/3/690.full.
69. BJ1., Boucher. Vitamin D insufficiency and diabetes risks. *PubMed*. [Online] Jan 2011.
https://www.ncbi.nlm.nih.gov/pubmed/20795936.
70. Asians., Glucose intolerance and impairment of insulin secretion in relation to vitamin
D deficiency in east London. Glucose intolerance and impairment of insulin secretion in
relation to vitamin D deficiency in east London Asians. *PubMed*. [Online] Oct 1995.
https://www.ncbi.nlm.nih.gov/pubmed/8690178.
71. Seyed A. Hoseini, Ashraf Aminorroaya, Bijan Iraj, and Massoud Amini. The effects of
oral vitamin D on insulin resistance in pre-diabetic patients. [Online] Jan 2013.
https://www.ncbi.nlm.nih.gov/pmc/articles/PMC3719226/.

72. Parildar H,Cigerli O, Unal DA, Gulmez O, and Demirag NG. The impact of Vitamin D Replacement on Glucose Metabolism. *PMC*. [Online] Nov 2013.
https://www.ncbi.nlm.nih.gov/pmc/articles/PMC3905396/.

73. Prue H. Hart, Shelley Gorman & John J. Finlay-Jones. Modulation of the immune system by UV radiation: more than just the effects of vitamin D? *Nature reviews IMMUNOLOGY.* [Online] Sep 2011.
http://www.nature.com/nri/journal/v11/n9/full/nri3045.html.

74. Masterjohn, Chris. Vitamin D is Synthesized From Cholesterol and Found in Cholesterol-Rich Foods. *Cholesterol and Health.* [Online] May 25, 2006.
http://www.cholesterol-and-health.com/Vitamin-D.html.

75. Schaefer, Anna and Kathryn Watson. What's the Relationship Between Vitamin D and Cholesterol? *Health Line.* [Online] Mar 2016. http://www.healthline.com/health/high-cholesterol/vitamin-d-relationship.

76. al, Cutillas-Marco E. et. https://www.ncbi.nlm.nih.gov/pmc/articles/PMC3908966/.
Vitamin D status and hypercholesterolemia in Spanish general population. [Online] PMC, Jun 2013. https://www.ncbi.nlm.nih.gov/pmc/articles/PMC3908966/.

77. Overbeck, Peter. Vitamin-D-Mangel geht aufs Herz. *ÄrzteZeitung.* [Online] Oct 12, 2012. http://www.aerztezeitung.de/medizin/krankheiten/herzkreislauf/article/823796/khk-infarkt-vitamin-d-mangel-geht-aufs-herz.html.

78. K, Nishio. *Nishio K, Mukae S, Aoki S, Itoh S, Konno N, Ozawa K, Satoh R, Katagiri T. Congestive heart failure is associated with the rate of bone loss. J Intern Med. Apr;253(4):439-46. 2003.* J Intern Med. Apr;253(4):439-46. 2003 : s.n., 2003.

79. Vitamin D bei Bluthochdruck? *Ärztezeitung.* [Online] May 14, 2012.
http://www.aerztezeitung.de/medizin/krankheiten/herzkreislauf/bluthochdruck/article/813149/vitamin-d-bluthochdruck.html.

80. Pilz, S., Iodice, S., Zittermann, A. et al. Vitamin D status and mortality risk in chronic kidney disease: a meta-analysis of prospective studies. *PubMed.* [Online] Sep 2011.
https://www.ncbi.nlm.nih.gov/pubmed/21636193.

81. Autier, P. & Gandini, S. *Vitamin D supplementation and total mortality: a meta-analysis of randomized controlled trials.* . Archives of Internal Medicine, 167, 1730–1737 : s.n., 2007.

82. Studie: Vitamin D Therapie Begleitende Vitamin D Therapie für IntensivpatientInnen erforscht. *Die Medizinische Universität Graz.* [Online]
https://www.medunigraz.at/neues/detail/news/studie-vitamin-d-therapie/.

83. Links between Vitamin D Deficiency and Cardiovascular Diseases. *PubMed.* [Online] Biomed Res Int. 2015; 2015: 109275.
https://www.ncbi.nlm.nih.gov/pmc/articles/PMC4427096/.

84. Kalkan GY1, Gür M2, Koyunsever NY1, Şeker T1, Gözükara MY3, Uçar H1, Kaypaklı O1, Baykan AO1, Akyol S1, Türkoğlu C1, Elbasan Z1, Şahin DY1, Çaylı M1. Serum 25-Hydroxyvitamin D Level and Aortic Intima-Media Thickness in Patients Without Clinical Manifestation of Atherosclerotic Cardiovascular Disease. *PubMed.* [Online] Jul 2015.
https://www.ncbi.nlm.nih.gov/pubmed/25130180.

85. Reusch, Sebastian. Wie entsteht Krebs? Ein vereinfachter Blick auf die Auslöser. *Spectrum Scilogs.* [Online] Mar 11, 2011. https://scilogs.spektrum.de/enkapsis/wie-entsteht-krebs-ein-vereinfachter-blick-auf-die-ausl-ser/.

86. Martinez ME, Giovannucci EL, Colditz GA, et al. Calcium, vitamin D, and the occurrence of colorectal cancer among women. J Natl Cancer Inst. 88:1375-1382. 1996. *PubMed.* [Online] https://www.ncbi.nlm.nih.gov/pmc/articles/PMC4545459/.

87. Salazar-Martinez E, Lazcano-Ponce EC, Gonzalez Lira-Lira G, Escudero-De los Rios P. Nutritional determinants of epithelial ovarian cancer risk: a case-control study in Mexico. Oncology. 63(2):151-7. 2002. *PubMed.* [Online] https://www.ncbi.nlm.nih.gov/pubmed/12239450.

88. Thys-Jacobs S, Donovan D, Papadopoulos A, et al. Vitamin D and calcium dysregulation in the polycystic ovarian syndrome. Steroids. 64:430-435. 1999. *PubMed.* [Online] https://www.ncbi.nlm.nih.gov/pubmed/10433180.

89. Cantorna M, Hayes C and DeLuca H. 1,25-Dihydroxycholecalciferol inhibits the progression of arthritis in murine models of human arthritis. Journal of Nutrition, v. 128, p. 68-72. 1998. *PubMed.* [Online] https://www.ncbi.nlm.nih.gov/pubmed/9430604.

90. Lemire J, Ince A and Takashima M. 1,25-dihydroxyvitamin D3 attenuates the expression of experimental murine lupus of MRL/l mice. Autoimmunity, v. 12, p. 143-148. 1992. *PubMed.* [Online] https://www.ncbi.nlm.nih.gov/pubmed/1617111.

91. Sharon L. McDonnell, Carole Baggerly, Christine B. French, Leo L. Baggerly, Cedric F. Garland, Edward D. Gorham, Joan M. Lappe, Robert P. Heaney. Serum 25-Hydroxyvitamin D Concentrations ≥40 ng/ml Are Associated with >65% Lower Cancer Risk: Pooled Analysis of Randomized Trial and Prospective Cohort Study. *PLOS ONE.* [Online] Apr 2016. http://journals.plos.org/plosone/article?id=10.1371/journal.pone.0152441.

92. Low Vitamin D Levels. *Breastcancer.org.* [Online] http://www.breastcancer.org/risk/factors/low_vit_d.

93. Esther, Kim. Lower Level Vitamin D During Remission Contributes To Relapse in Ulcerative Colitis Patients. *Beth Israel Deaconess Medical Center.* [Online] Feb 17, 2017. http://www.bidmc.org/News/PRLandingPage/2017/February/Moss-Ulcerative-Colitis-Vitamin-D.aspx.

94. Peterson, Riley. Recent study finds that low vitamin D levels are associated with increased disease activity in ulcerative colitis. *Vitamin D Council.* [Online] Jul 14, 2016. https://www.vitamindcouncil.org/recent-study-finds-that-low-vitamin-d-levels-are-associated-with-increased-disease-activity-in-ulcerative-colitis/.

95. Ladegaard, Isak. Cancer patients with high vitamin D levels live longer. *Science Nordic.* [Online] Aug 15, 2012. http://sciencenordic.com/cancer-patients-high-vitamin-d-levels-live-longer.

96. Dima A Youssef,1,2 Christopher WT Miller,3 Adel M El-Abbassi,1,2 Della C Cutchins,1 Coleman Cutchins,5 William B Grant,4 and Alan N Peiriscorresponding author1,2. Antimicrobial implications of vitamin D. *Dermato Endocrinology.* [Online] Oct 2011. https://www.ncbi.nlm.nih.gov/pmc/articles/PMC3256336/.

97. Garland, Dr. Cedric. Vitamin D & Premenopausal Breast Cancer – Deficiency Increases Risk. *GrassrootsHealth.* [Online] http://www.grassrootshealth.net/garlandbctranscription.

98. Nonclassic Actions of Vitamin D. *Oxford academic.* [Online] Jan 2009. https://academic.oup.com/jcem/article-lookup/doi/10.1210/jc.2008-1454.

99. Paddock, Catharine PhD. Cancer risk falls with higher levels of vitamin D. *Medical News Today.* [Online] Apr 8, 2016. http://www.medicalnewstoday.com/articles/308834.php.

100. Wagner, Carol L, Sarah N Taylor, Donna D Johnson, and Bruce W Hollis. The role of vitamin D in pregnancy and lactation: emerging concepts. *PMC.* [Online] 2012. https://www.ncbi.nlm.nih.gov/pmc/articles/PMC4365424/.

101. VITAMIN D IN DER SCHWANGERSCHAFT. [Online] http://www.vitamind.net/schwangerschaft/.

102. Pregnancy and gestational vitamin D deficiency. *Vitamin D Council.* [Online] 2015. https://www.vitamindcouncil.org/newsletter-pregnancy-and-gestational-vitamin-d-deficiency/.

103. Bodnar LM1, Krohn MA, Simhan HN. Maternal vitamin D deficiency is associated with bacterial vaginosis in the first trimester of pregnancy. *PubMed.* [Online] Jun 2009. https://www.ncbi.nlm.nih.gov/pubmed/19357214.

104. Lapillonne, A. Vitamin D deficiency during pregnancy may impair maternal and fetal outcomes. *Med Hypotheses .* [Online] Jan 2010. https://www.ncbi.nlm.nih.gov/pubmed/19692182.

105. Lee V1, Rekhi E, Hoh Kam J, Jeffery G. Vitamin D rejuvenates aging eyes by reducing inflammation, clearing amyloid beta and improving visual function. *PubMed.* [Online] Oct 2012. https://www.ncbi.nlm.nih.gov/pubmed/22217419.

106. Conin, Joseph. Vitamin D Reportedly Improves Vision. *opticalceu.blogspot.* [Online] Jan 2012. http://opticalceu.blogspot.ch/2012/01/vitamin-d-reportedly-improves-vision.html.

107. Bates, Claire. Boosting vitamin D levels 'could help prevent eyesight from deteriorating'. *Mail Online.* [Online] Jan 2012. Boosting vitamin D levels 'could help prevent eyesight from deteriorating.

108. Martens, Dd.phil. Alexander. Sportler brauchen Vitamin D. *http://www.irmgard-graef.de/.* [Online] Jul 2017. http://www.irmgard-graef.de/neue-studien/vitamin-d/sportler-brauchen-vitamin-d/.

109. Cannell, John. *Athlets Edge - Faster, Quicker, Tronger.* s.l. : Here and Now, 2011. ISBN 978-0-9774272-9-1.

110. Fautek, Dr. Jan-Dirk. *Melatonin DAs Geheimnis eines wunderbaren Hormons.* Wien : Brandstetter, 2017. ISBN 978-3-7106-0056-2.

111. Editor. Pineal Gland Calcification. *The Event Chronicle.* [Online] Dec 7, 2015. http://www.theeventchronicle.com/metaphysics/metascience/pineal-gland-calcification-why-you-should-care/.

112. Allemann, Sarha. ETH empfiehlt noch höhere Vitamin-D-Zufuhr. *SRF PLUS.* [Online] ec 1, 2015. https://www.srf.ch/sendungen/puls/koerper/eth-empfiehlt-noch-hoehere-vitamin-d-zufuhr.

113. Holick, Michael PHD. VITAMIN D: A D-LIGHTFUL SOLUTION FOR HEALTH. *PMC.* [Online] Aug 2011. https://www.ncbi.nlm.nih.gov/pmc/articles/PMC3738435/.

114. Boucher, Barbara J. The Problems of Vitamin D Insufficiency in Older People. *PMC.* [Online] Aug 2012. https://www.ncbi.nlm.nih.gov/pmc/articles/PMC3501367/.

115. Fuchs, Marita. Gesund bleiben mit Vitamin D. *Universität Zürich.* [Online] Dec 18, 2012. http://www.news.uzh.ch/de/articles/2012/dreierpack-fuer-gesundes-altern.html.

116. A new look at vitamin D challenges the current view of its benefits. [Online] Oct 2016. http://www.buckinstitute.org/buck-news/new-look-vitamin-d-challenges-current-view-its-benefits.

117. Podbregar, Nadja. Das Geheimnis der Telomere Altern und die Rolle der Chromosomen-Endkappen. *scinexx.de Das Wissensmagazin.* [Online] Apr 16, 2010. http://www.scinexx.de/dossier-detail-490-6.html.

118. Mamtani, Mira. *(R)EVOLUTION IM ANTI-AGING: DIE WISSENSCHAFT DER TELOMERE.* 2016. ISBN 978-3-96051-520-3.

119. Mohsen Mazidi, corresponding author1,2 Erin D. Michos,3,4 and Maciej Banach5,6. The association of telomere length and serum 25-hydroxyvitamin D levels in US adults: the National Health and Nutrition Examination Survey. *PMC.* [Online] Feb 1, 2017. https://www.ncbi.nlm.nih.gov/pmc/articles/PMC5206371/.

120. Murnaghan, Ian BSc (hons), MS. An Overview of DNA Functions. [Online] Jan 2017. http://www.exploredna.co.uk/an-overview-dna-functions.html.

121. James C. Fleet, 1,5 Marsha DeSmet,4 Robert Johnson,2 and Yan Li3. Vitamin D and Cancer: A review of molecular mechanisms. *HHS Public Access.* [Online] Sep 2015. https://www.ncbi.nlm.nih.gov/pmc/about/public-access/.

122. Nair-Shalliker V, Armstrong BK, Fenech M. Does vitamin D protect against DNA damage? *PubMed .* [Online] May 2012. https://www.ncbi.nlm.nih.gov/pubmed/22366026.

123. Gräf, Irmgard Maria. *Mein Blut - ein Weg zu mir.* Peiting : Miachels Verlag, 20147. ISBN 978-3895-398-988.

124. Bunzel, Tom. www.collective-evolution.com. *As Above So Below: What Can Other Or Higher "Dimensions" Really Mean?* [Online] https://www.collective-evolution.com/2015/09/18/as-above-so-below-what-can-other-or-higher-dimensions-really-mean/.

125. Pollack, H Gerald. *Fourth Phase of Water; Beyond Solid, Liquid & Vapor.* s.l. : Ebner & Sons Publishers, 2013. 978-0962689543.

126. Decker, Jerry. Dr. Pollack and the case for a Fourth phase of water. . [Online] Jun 2015. https://atlantisrisingmagazine.com/article/dr-pollack-and-the-case-for-a-fourth-phase-of-water/.

127. Water. [Online] 2005. http://www.whatthebleep.com/water-crystals/.

128. Ultraviolettstrahlung. *Welt der Physik.* [Online] March 2006. http://www.weltderphysik.de/gebiet/atome/elektromagnetisches-spektrum/ultraviolettstrahlung/.

129. Rowen, Robert Jay. The Cure that Time forgot - Ultraviolet Blood Irradiation Therapy (Photo-Oxidation). *Foundation For Biosocial Research.* [Online] 1996. http://www.vitamind.arcarmichael.com/Irradiation/rowen.htm.

130. Tesla coil. [Online] https://en.wikipedia.org/wiki/Tesla_coil.

131. Brown Tom. Tesla Coil - Lost Inventions of Nikola Tesla. [Online] http://altered-states.net/barry/newsletter208/.

132. UV Light Part III Photoluminescence Therapy. [Online] 2006. http://www.mnwelldir.org/docs/uv_light/uv_light3.htm.

133. Havasi, Peter. *Education of Cancer Healing Vol. VII-Heretics.* s.l. : Lulu, 2012. ISBN: 978-1-291-45368-3.

134. Campell, William Douglas II, MD. *Into the Light, Tomorrows medicine Today.* Panama City : Rhino Publishing , 1993, 2003. ISBN 9962-636-27-2.

135. ST. PETERSBURG UPGRADES WATER TREATMENT PLANTS WITH UV SYSTEMS. [Online] http://www.waterworld.com/articles/wwi/print/volume-20/issue-10/features/st-petersburg-upgrades-water-treatment-plants-with-uv-systems.html.

136. UV Lights to Sanitize a St. Petersburg Air Conditioner. [Online] 2006. https://de.scribd.com/document/233875106/UV-Lights-to-Sanitize-a-St-Petersburg-Air-Conditioner.

137. empa, Six, Andrea. Leucht Pyjama für Neugeborene. *ww.empa.ch/web/s604/photonic-textiles-for-newborns.* [Online] Nov 05, 2017. ww.empa.ch/web/s604/photonic-textiles-for-newborns.

138. Minguillon, Jesus, Miguel Angel Lopez-Gordo, Diego A. Renedo-Criado, Maria Jose Sanchez-Carrion, Francisco Pelayo. Blue lighting accelerates post-stress relaxation: Results of a preliminary study. [Online] 2017. http://journals.plos.org/plosone/article?id=10.1371/journal.pone.0186399.

139. *Leistung: Schneller dank blauem Licht.* 20.05.2017, St. Gallen : St. Galler Tagblatt, 2017.

140. Shirazian, Shayan, Olufemi Aina, Youngjun Park, Nawsheen Chowdhury,1 Kathleen Leger, Linle Hou, Nobuyuki Miyawaki, and Vandana S Mathur. Chronic kidney disease-associated pruritus: impact on quality of life and current management challenges. *PMC.* [Online] Jan 2017. https://www.ncbi.nlm.nih.gov/pmc/articles/PMC5271405/.

141. https://www.nau.ch/politik/forschung/2018/07/05/blaues-licht-hilft-in-spateren-stadien-der-wundheilung-65364067. [Online] 2018.

142. *Neue Technologien für die Medizin.* s.l. : arte TV, 2018. https://www.arte.tv/de/videos/078767-001-A/neue-technologien-fuer-die-medizin/.

143. Schindler, Michael. When the Pills Don't Help: Finding Your Way-Forward. [Online] Jun 2017. http://blog.seattlepi.com/militarywire/2017/06/19/when-the-pills-dont-help-finding-your-way-forward/.

144. Venefica, Avia. Symbolic meaning of Octagon. *symbolic meanings.* [Online] May 2008. http://www.symbolic-meanings.com/2008/05/24/symbolic-meaning-of-octagon/.

145. The origin of time and the secret of nine. *Trace Elements Radio.* [Online] 2015. http://www.traceelementsradio.com/2015/12/the-origin-of-time-and-secret-of-nine.html.

146. Wolf, Christopher and Mohammad R. K. Mofrad. PMC National library. *On the Octagonal Structure of the Nuclear Pore Complex: Insights from Coarse-Grained Models.* [Online] May 2008. https://www.ncbi.nlm.nih.gov/pmc/articles/PMC2483776/.

147. Tom Kenyon. *Erneuerung.* [Online] Feb 2017. http://tomkenyon.com/erneuerung.

148. Pelkowski, Udo. FREQUENZEN - Der Ursprung , sowie die verändernde Kraft allen Lebens. *Alles im Universum ist Schwingung.* [Online] Aug 17, 2013.

https://www.facebook.com/notes/anneliese-m%C3%BCller/frequenzen-der-ursprung-sowie-die-ver%C3%A4ndernde-kraft-allen-lebens/521524107917778/.

149. Horowitz, Dr. Leonard G. *Healing Codes - Biological Apocalypse.* s.l. : Medical Veritas International; Auflage: Reprint (Mai 1999), 1999. ISBN-13: 978-0923550394.

150. The Sacred Solfeggio Frequencies. [Online] http://www.warrior-priestess.com/12strandDNA-Solfeggio.html.

151. Gehirnwellen und Gehirnwellenbereiche. *i-NFBF.* [Online] http://www.i-nfbf.ch/de/gehirnwellen.html.

152. What are Brainwaves. *brainworks.* [Online] http://www.brainworksneurotherapy.com/what-are-brainwaves.

153. Learn about the Wonders of Theta Medidation Music. *Binaural Beats Medidation.* [Online] https://www.binauralbeatsmeditation.com/the-wonders-of-theta-meditation-music/.

154. The Benefits of Gamma Brainwaves. *Brainwave Wizard.* [Online] http://brainwavewizard.com/entrainment/the-benefits-of-gamma-brainwaves/.

155. https://www.i-nfbf.ch/de/gehirnwellen.html. [Online]

156. Bortfeldt, Dr. Kerstin. http://instatera.de/das-geheimnis-der-mikrotubuli-teil-i/. [Online] 2017.

157. Petros C. Benias, Rebecca G. Wells, Bridget Sackey-Aboagye, Heather Klavan, Jason Reidy, Darren Buonocore, Markus Miranda, Susan Kornacki, Michael Wayne, David L. Carr-Locke & Neil D. Theise . Scientific Reports. *Structure and Distribution of an Unrecognized Interstitium in Human Tissues.* [Online] Mar 27, 2018. https://www.nature.com/articles/s41598-018-23062-6.

158. Pollack, Dr. Gerald. *Wasser - viel mehr als H2O.* Kirchzarten : VAK Verlag GmbH, 2013/2015. ISBN 978-3-86731-158-8.

159. Briner, Lindsay. Neurohacker Collective. [Online] https://neurohacker.com/people/lindsay-briner.

160. Photonentherapie nach Prof. Popp. [Online] 1999. https://www.dr-neidert.de/therapien/photonentherapie.

161. Bertone, Nikki. Nikki Bertones Story. [Online] Jan 2017. http://bluroom.com/emailers/0123_NWS/online_STY.html.

162. Ein besonderer Fall- Erosive Osteochondrose verschwunden. *Instatera Blu Room Weimar.* [Online] Jul 13, 2016. http://instatera.de/ein-besonderer-fall-erosive-osteochondrose/.

163. http://bluroomwellnesscenter.com/testimonials/. [Online] 2017. http://bluroomwellnesscenter.com/testimonials/.

164. https://www.facebook.com/BluRoomCH/posts/blu-room-und-hyperthyreose-schilddr%C3%BCsenutnerfunkt/882316755252719/. [Online] 2017.

165. http://bluroomwellnesscenter.com/news/. *Blu Room Wellness Center.* [Online] 2018. http://bluroomwellnesscenter.com/news/.

166. Bortfeldt, Dr. Kerstin, Pirker, Dr. Andrea. *Vom KrankSein und GesundSein.* s.l. : book on demand, 2017. ISBN 9783746031569.

167. Gräf, Irmgard Maria. *Die Quark-Öl-Kur. Die Heilkraft der Öl-Eiweiss-Ernährung nach Dr. Budwig.* s.l. : Verlag Vianova, 2014 .

168. —. Mein Blut - ein Weg zu mir. Peiting : Michaels Verlag, 2014.

169. —. *Blu Room - Experience the future. Building bridges with light, frequency and sound.* Yelm : Blu Room Enterprises, 2017. ISBN 9781547129157.

170. —. *Die Blaue Quelle - Theorie und Potenzial der Blu Room Technologie.* s.l. : book on demand, 2018. ISBN 9783752848137.

171. Wesley, J. Pike, Ph.D. and Mark B. Meyer, Ph.D. The Vitamin D Receptor: New Paradigms for the Regulation of Gene Expression by 1,25-Dihydroxyvitamin D3. *PMC.* [Online] Jan 2011. https://www.ncbi.nlm.nih.gov/pmc/articles/PMC2879406/.

172. LeBlanc ES, Rizzo JH, Pedula KL, Ensrud KE, Cauley J, Hochberg M, Hillier TA and Fractures., Study Of Osteoporotic. Associations between 25-hydroxyvitamin D and weight gain in elderly women. *VitaminDWiki.* [Online] Dec 2012. http://www.vitamindwiki.com/tiki-index.php?page_id=3551.

173. Engelman, Corinne. Vitamin D may block the obesity gene FTO. *VitaminDWiki .* [Online] Feb 2014. http://www.vitamindwiki.com/Vitamin+D+may+block+the+obesity+gene+%28FTO%29+%E2%80%93+Jan+2014.

174. Reichrath, Jörg, Bodo Lehmann, Jörg Spitz. *Vitamin D update 2012 Von der Rachitisprophylaxe zur allgemeinen Gesundheitsvorsorge.* München : Dustri Verlag, 2012.

175. Mark, Karla PhD. A new look at vitamin D challenges the current view of its benefits. *buckinstitute.* [Online] Oct 2016. http://www.buckinstitute.org/buck-news/new-look-vitamin-d-challenges-current-view-its-benefits.

176. Ramtha. *Das Gehirn: Schöpfer von Realität und einem erhabenen Leben.* s.l. : Gabriel Reinert ligvid.media, 2015. ISBN-13: 978-3940786593.

177. The Law of Vibration. *One Mind - One energy.* [Online] http://www.one-mind-one-energy.com/Law-of-vibration.html.

178. The Law of Vibration. [Online] http://www.natural-health-zone.com/law-of-vibration.html.

179. *Blut - Highway des Lebens.* Gräf. s.l. : Matrix3000, Vol. 86.

180. Sills, Franklin. *The Breath of Life, Holism and Biodynamics.* Berkeley CA : North Atlantic Books, 2011.

181. Coats, Callum. *Naturenergien verstehen und nutzen.* Aachen : Omega, 2001. ISBN 3-930243-14-8.

182. Vitamin, D the "sunshine" vitamin. Vitamin D: The "sunshine" vitamin. *PMC.* [Online] Apr 2012. https://www.ncbi.nlm.nih.gov/pmc/articles/PMC3356951/.

183. United States Patent. *https://patents.justia.com/patent/9919162.* [Online] Mar 20, 2018.

184. Dürr, Prof. Dr. Hans-Peter. *Wir erleben mehr als wir begreifen - Naturwissenschaftliche -Erkenntnis und Erleben der Wirklichkeit.* [https://www.youtube.com/watch?v=oVEQoUynYHk] 2002.

185. Fosar, G., F. Bludorf. *Vernetzte Intelligenz.* s.l. : Omega, 2006. ISBN-13: 978-3930243235.

186. Gräf, Irmgard Maria. *Blu Room - Zukunft hautnah erleben.* Maienfeld : s.n., 2017. ISBN 9781547129157.

INDEX

spinal cord · 50
stability · 35, 65, 90, 97
stem cell · 97
stress · 25, 39, 45, 70, 84, 94, 101, 103
sunlight · 16, 18, 19, 21, 29, 34, 37, 42, 49, 57, 96

T

telomere · 68, 97, 99
Tesla, Nikola · 28, 80
The Blue Fountain · 113
thyroid · 38, 57, 104
toxins · 25, 46, 66, 81, 98
trauma · 70, 97, 104

U

ulcerative colitis · 61

UVA frequency · 19, 20
UVB frequency · 6, 19, 20, 26, 37, 43, 44, 56, 78, 80, 84, 85, 88, 90, 96, 98
UVB-frequency · 20
UVC frequency · 20, 84

V

Vitamin D · 5, 6, 16, 17, 18, 20, 35, 37, 38, 39, 40, 41, 42, 43, 44, 45, 46, 47, 48, 49, 50, 51, 53, 54, 55, 56, 57, 58, 59, 60, 61, 62, 63, 64, 65, 66, 67, 68, 69, 70, 96, 97
Vitamin D receptor · 37

W

wound healing · 84, 85, 105